EXTREME FITNESS

Skyhorse Publishing books may be purchased in bulk at special discounts for sales
promotion, corporate gifts, fund-raising, or educational purposes. Special editions
can also be created to specifications. For details, contact the Special Sales Department, Skyhorse Publishing, 307 West 36th Street, 11th Floor, New York, NY 10018 or
info@skyhorsepublishing.com.

Skyhorse® and Skyhorse Publishing® are registered trademarks of
Skyhorse Publishing, Inc.®, a Delaware corporation.

www.skyhorsepublishing.com

10 9 8 7 6 5 4 3 2 1

Library of Congress Cataloging-in-Publication Data is available on file.

Cover design by Brian Peterson
Cover images by Per Bernal
Skyhorse edition edited by Constance Renfrow

Paperback ISBN: 978-1-5107-5520-8
Ebook ISBN: 978-1-62914-925-7

Printed in China

EXTREME
FITNESS

HOW TO TRAIN LIKE
AN ACTION HERO

DOLPH LUNDGREN

Photography by Per Bernal
Translated by Brandon Schultz

SKYHORSE PUBLISHING

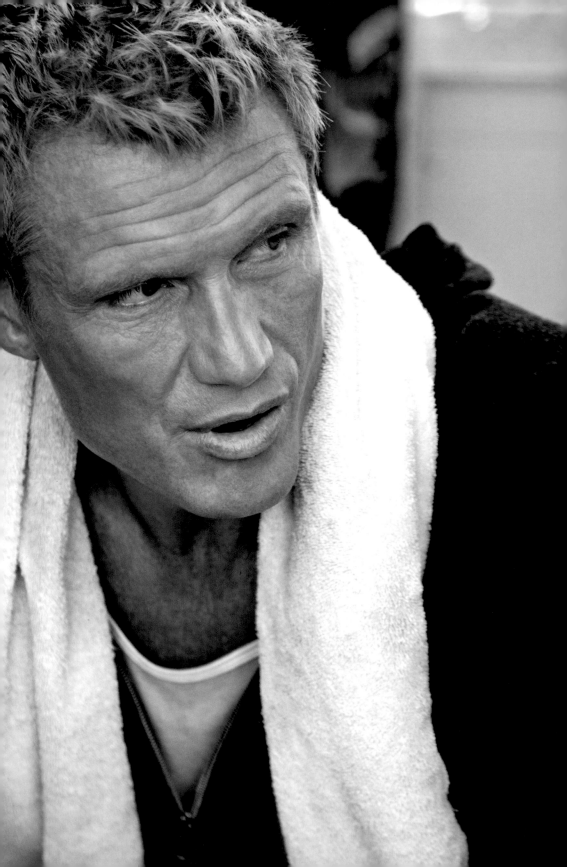

CONTENTS

Much has happened since I first considered writing a book on physical fitness. The original title *Fit at Forty* referred to the period when I lived in New York City in the late '90s.

My body was beat after a year of non-stop filming. I flirted with the idea of taking a break from Hollywood to get my third-degree black belt in karate. Taking the elevator down to 64th Street, I jogged across Lexington Avenue to my favorite gym to gather my thoughts during a workout.

I didn't write the book then. A few years later, I earned my third *Dan* black belt during a tough grading. The manila folder with book ideas disappeared into a dusty cabinet. At some point I changed the handwritten title on the front to *Fit 4-Ever*.

As always my friends and family kept asking me for advice on diet and exercise. My desire to write the book was still there, smoldering under the surface.

Fast-forward to ten years later. I was asked to be a host of a radio show back in my home country of Sweden. The format of this popular summer program is that the host to talks about a specific topic of his or her choice for ninety minutes, interspersed with music. I decided to talk about my dad. During an emotional live broadcast, I relived my childhood's tears and joy. After being away from Sweden for so long, I realized how important it was to me to finally feel understood and embraced by my fellow countrymen. The memories of that afternoon broadcast still make me choke up.

Because of the reaction to this broadcast, the idea of writing a book about my life and my adventures in Hollywood was brought forward by a number of Swedish publishers. One publisher mentioned another idea: a fitness book. I thought about it. Instead of writing a traditional biography or an exercise manual, the result was an autobiographical fitness book. As one comedian put it, "I knocked up two birds with one stone."

I decided to write a book not only filled with personal training advice, but one that also tries to explain how physical training literally saved my life as a teenager and later became an unshakable part of it.

"A healthy man has many wishes. The sick man only one," says an old Indian proverb. Life is a gift for us to enjoy. A strong body is essential for good health. Without our health, we cannot fully experience the wonderful world around us.

The fact that my book is now being published in the United States makes the whole experience so much sweeter. Everything I've accomplished in the past thirty years has happened because I decided to come to America. The first act of my story takes place in Scandinavia, but the more exciting parts happen across the Atlantic.

So, very fittingly, I sit here in a hotel suite in Los Angeles finishing the manuscript for my book. Tomorrow at 5:30 a.m., I'll be in the hotel gym with a pair of dumbbells in my hands.

C'est la vie . . .

I sincerely hope that physical fitness will be as important a part of your life as it has been in mine.

/ West Hollywood, April, 2014

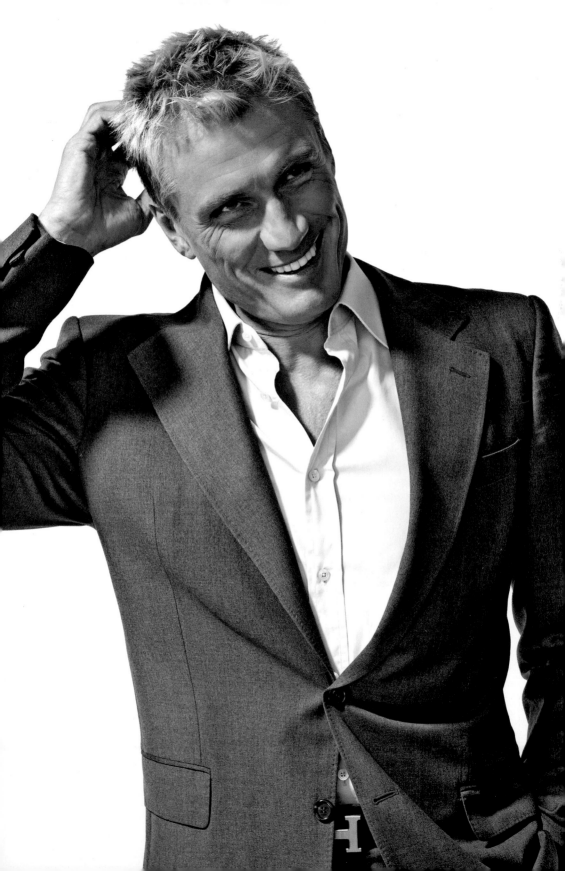

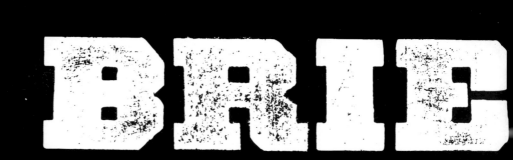

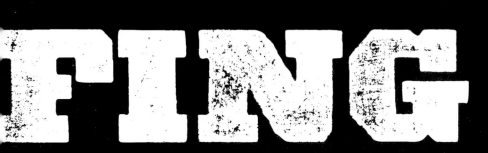

TRAIN TO LIVE—AND SURVIVE

Life can sometimes feel like a movie that's too long, where the characters and story don't make sense. Remember that it's your life and you can write your own script. You can always choose to change yourself, to seek out new paths for a more harmonious and joyful life.

The choice is yours here and now. After all, you're the star of your own life. Play it well and enjoy the movie.

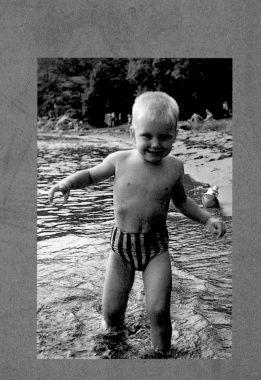

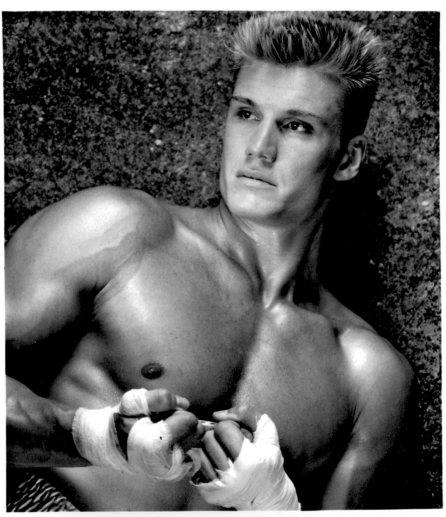

"ROCKY IV"

from

MGM/UA Entertainment Co.

R-38 **DOLPH LUNDGREN** (Above) stars as Ivan Drago, a 6'6", 240 pound Soviet fighting machine known as "the Siberian Express" — the deadliest opponent Rocky Balboa has ever faced in the ring.

PHOTO CREDIT: E.J. Camp.

Left: A very young Ivan Drago

It may be hard to believe, but the super athlete Ivan Drago wasn't the athletic type during his childhood or early adolescence. On the contrary, I was "morbidly weak," as they say up in the grim northern Swedish provinces.

"You who are small and weak must go to the Salvation Army Hall. I who am big and strong will go party and have a ball!" said my Swedish uncle Sture, an amateur boxer and amateur comedian. He grinned and unbuttoned his shirt, flexing his hairy, muscular chest.

One of my earliest blurry childhood memories is from a hospital in Stockholm. I remember the dim lights and the smells. Ether vapors, disinfectants, or whatever it may have been. I lay alone in my hospital room staring up at the ceiling. As a four-year-old, I had croup, a viral disease of the respiratory tract that resulted in an acute shortness of breath. Later, my parents told me that they thought I would die when my face turned blue and I couldn't breathe. After this disease, "Little Hans," as I was called at the time, developed persistent allergies and asthma. I wasn't allowed to be outside playing with the other kids. My eyes were swollen in the summer and I had to walk around with a black pirate patch, holding in place a cotton ball soaked in boric acid. I kept moving the patch from one eye to the other depending on which eye hurt the most. Half asleep, my mother would stay up with me through the night when I had my asthma attacks and couldn't breathe.

The asthma affected my physical and emotional development. I could play simple kids' games, but I couldn't participate in any organized sports. Instead, I ended up focusing on wimpy indoor activities like music and painting. I suffered during both my grade school and junior high school PE classes. When it was time to pick teams, I was almost always chosen last. Just ahead of some girl with no athletic talent to speak of.

I became a target for bullying from the bigger boys at school.

These are memories that I carried with me for some time. The good news was that, even though I was unaware of it at the time, I had started to build up a need for affirmation and comeback. This inner strength would be of great help to me later in life.

Have you decided to invest in exercise? Congratulations. You've made a decision that will make you feel better both physically and mentally. If you're not used to regular exercise, you'll be surprised how quickly your body responds to it. If you're already exercising regularly, you'll know that the human body was created to move and it feels good to get it moving. Human beings are extremely adaptable. Not just in relation to the environment, but also in relation to themselves. Homo sapiens have survived as a species because we have a tremendous ability to change.

When you decide to change something in your life, for instance your exercise habits, you need to understand why you want that change. Only then can you achieve a lasting change. Lasting change should be the goal of any major effort we make in our lives.

Getting in shape is not only about making the clothes in your closet fit a little better. Looking good at the beach. Being able to lift heavier weights at the gym. Sure, these positive effects may be goals, but they're actually just perks that come with the territory. Understanding why you need to get in shape is more important. This knowledge gives a real meaning to your training. Once you understand your overall goals, prioritizing your training regimen will become easier.

For me, physical fitness is both a reward and a source of energy. It builds my physique, but it also

> "YOU WHO ARE SMALL AND WEAK MUST GO TO THE SALVATION ARMY HALL. I WHO AM BIG AND STRONG WILL PARTY AND HAVE A BALL!" SAID MY SWEDISH UNCLE STURE. HE GRINNED AND UNBUTTONED HIS SHIRT, FLEXING HIS HAIRY, MUSCULAR CHEST.

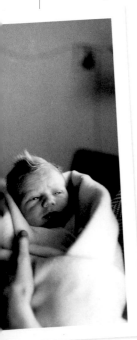

A newborn Hans Dolph Lundgren

increases my mental focus. Training has been part of my life for so long that it would be difficult for me to function without it. I might be able to survive physically, but it would be harder to go on mentally.

In my youth, it was precisely through sports and training that I found myself. I realized that I too had the ability to accomplish something special with my life. As a young boy, it wasn't just in the schoolyard that I felt like a loser. It was even tougher on the home front.

My father was a well-educated engineer, army officer, and high-ranking government official. He was also manic depressive, sometimes bordering on schizophrenic. He had a volatile temper that was extremely unpredictable, to put it mildly.

I believe that his emotional outbreaks came in response to his—in his own eyes—unfulfilling and failed career. Without warning, he could flare up and become extremely violent. He took out his inner frustrations on me and on my mom with a vengeance. With fists, boots, my soccer shoes, rolled-up newspapers, and any other weapon that happened to be in the general vicinity.

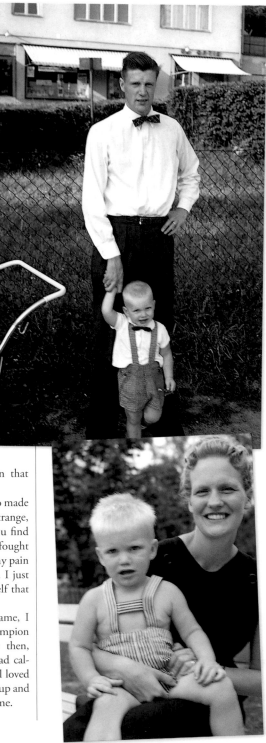

These assaults hurt me physically, but also made me shut down emotionally. It may sound strange, but you can get used to physical abuse. You find strategies to survive and even retaliate. I fought back by trying not to scream, cry, or show any pain when he hit me. I wasn't always successful. I just lay there, took the pain, and swore to myself that one day I would be able fight back.

But years later when that day finally came, I couldn't do it. I was a black-belt karate champion and strong enough to take him on. By then, Director K. H. Lundgren, (MSc, MBA), had calmed down emotionally. And somehow I still loved and respected my father. I couldn't just walk up and slug him in the jaw for what he had done to me.

With Mom and Dad

14

The psychological damage done to me during those years was actually worse than the physical pain. This probably holds true for most similar childhood experiences. When my dad had his dark periods, he would tell me that I was worthless and that I would never become anything good. My self-esteem deteriorated further because I could not protect my own mother from his violent outbursts. To me this was yet another confirmation that I was a useless weakling who couldn't do anything right.

Of course, my childhood wasn't all bad news. Things got better when I slowly recovered from my allergies and asthma. I started jogging around the block, adding a loop a week, to strengthen my weak lungs.

One day, as an eleven-year-old, I noticed a colorful ad in a weekly magazine. It featured a picture of slick-haired Swedish strong man Arne Tammer, who flexed his huge biceps and declared: "Give me fifteen minutes a day and I will give you a new body!" This was the Scandinavian version of "The Bully of the Beach" campaign with Charles Atlas. I immediately ordered a twelve-week course and eagerly began training in our kitchen with my best buddies. Push-ups,

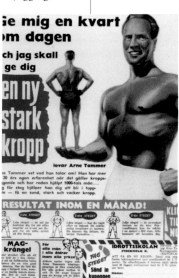

sit-ups, and squats were the exercises that we used to beef up our pale, scrawny bodies. We rushed like mad through an obstacle course we had constructed behind our suburban home.

Through my supreme effort and tears I gained a new insight: I hated to lose.

In those days, fitness training was an unfamiliar term to the common man. Yes, there was the odd "strong man" who lifted weights. People played classic Swedish sports like soccer and hockey. The average person was in pretty good shape. Daily exercise was a natural part of one's life. Not something that people discussed or read books about.

For a teenager in the sixties and seventies, exercise was just a natural part of one's day. Video games had not yet been invented and parents woke their kids up on weekends with the order, "Go outside and play!" I would happily walk or cycle five miles daily, sometimes longer, to go to school or visit friends. The diet was also different. I was lucky to enjoy one Coca-Cola once a month as a child. Later, as a somewhat more privileged teenager, I was allowed perhaps one Coke a week.

Today, a sedentary life in front of laptops and TVs have become the norm for most young people. More and more alarming reports about obesity, diabetes, and depression among our youth appear in the media. It's not that I believe the younger generation should immediately go out *en masse* to start playing sports and lifting weights. However, a better understanding and a greater awareness of physical activity and exercise are necessary to reverse a disturbing trend. What we lack today in the form of natural physical activity, we can compensate for with regular and varied physical training.

You might think that all this sounds a bit extreme, coming from a fitness fanatic who doesn't do much more than staying in shape for action scenes on the silver screen and glamorous appearances with beautiful women on the red carpet.

"Hey! Of course Dolph has to exercise regularly! His various movie roles require it. His whole career's built on looking fit and being tough. It's easy for him to take time out to train. His life is nothing like the average guy's."

Okay, living and working in my world may be different compared to many people, but my attitude toward exercise has to do with much more than being an actor.

Ask yourself what physical training and sports mean to you, in your life. Is it something you do just for the summer's first beach visit? When you look a bit too chubby in the mirror? To be less out of breath when you climb the stairs to your office? Or have you made physical exercise an integral part of your life?

If I had to prioritize the things that I value in my life, it would look something like this:

1. The health and happiness of my family
The first priority, a feeling I share with anybody who experiences the joy of becoming a parent or having a partner they love.

2. My own health and happiness
Without mental and physical health, it's very difficult to have a fulfilling life and to help others.

3. Self-realization through work and new challenges
It is important that you like what you do for a living. You have to feel a burning passion for something in order to do it really well.

4. Money
Is important, but comes last on my list. There is nothing wrong with building a fortune, but chasing money should never be an end in itself. Money can provide comfort and freedom. It can't buy you happiness, love, or health.

How often do you look at your life this way? All of us should sometimes look at our life's priorities. I try to do it every day.

In the United States, there is a strong focus on money and success. We are constantly reminded of the American Dream—especially in the entertainment industry, where I work. The image of a country that gives everybody the equal opportunity to achieve success and prosperity is what the New World was built on. As long as you have a dream and are willing to work damn hard to make it happen, you can achieve anything.

Points 3 and 4 from my setup above ("work" and "money") start sneaking in, trying to take over the spotlight. I sometimes lose sight of my own principles. To prevent this, I try to keep track of my workload and periodically remind myself not to get carried away with it and lose the control of

my own time. It is not always that simple. Believe me, there is no end to how hard you can work in Hollywood. There are always new projects and roles to aspire to. Promotional and publicity appearances are right there when you're not busy filming. We want to do it all. I made the same mistake when I first got into the business. And still do sometimes.

The film and TV industry is very seductive when you're in the zone and success is on your side. It's easy to believe that you have the energy to stand in front of the camera from early morning until late at night. Doing this day in and day out, month after month. Unfortunately it can cost more than it's worth, unless you know how to take care of yourself. The fear of being replaced and becoming a "has-been" are incredibly strong in this industry.

Working too hard without a break is the biggest oversight that many people commit. The first priority away from a time-pressed agenda should be proper exercise, food, and rest. We have to show a real consideration for our own health. Forgetting this is a big mistake, especially in the entertainment industry. If you're out of shape or aren't feeling on top, it shows very quickly. Serious consequences result when you don't look your best, particularly in Hollywood. Well, unless you got out of shape intentionally for that award-winning character role.

Open a decade-old magazine and see how many of the celebrities are still popular today. Some of the former stars are so out of shape and have aged to such a degree that you can hardly believe you are looking at the same person.

In summation: No matter how you look at it, it's always smart to invest extra time to physical exercise, relaxation, and recuperation. You'll have more energy available for other things you want to do.

The situation with my dad was difficult when I was a young boy, grabbing at straws to find my own identity. Most kids love their parents unconditionally, regardless of how they are treated. It was tough to be beaten by somebody you admire. Abused by someone from whom you want emotional support, love, and approval. The situation was hugely frustrating and confusing for a young boy like Hans Lundgren in the Stockholm city suburbs in the sixties.

To make things more complicated, I looked up to and admired my dad in many ways. On many occasions my father, Karl-Hugo, could be very funny, extremely charming, intelligent, and resourceful. He never drank too much and always dressed in impeccably tailored English suits, shirt and tie, wearing an exclusive aftershave. "Your dad looks like 'The Saint,'" remarked one girl at school. This was around the time when British actor Roger Moore, later James Bond, became famous as the suave crime-fighter "The Saint." (A funny sidenote is that many years later I would appear in one of his films, also dressed in suit and tie). One reason my dad looked so saintly was probably because my mom stayed with him throughout her entire adult life, obediently following orders until the day she prematurely passed away at the age of sixty. Worn out from waiting on him hand and foot.

Later in life, I've come to realize that my dad fought a constant battle with his own inner demons and damaged self-image. This was probably due to the abuse that he was subjected to by his own parents. He grew up during the economic depression of the 1930s. This was a time when poor people still starved to death in rural Sweden. Exactly what was done to him as a child is still a mystery. He kept that to himself.

My dad was 6'4" (exactly as tall as me) and had a massive interest in sports, particularly cross-country skiing, running, and the rusty barbell down in the basement. I guess he found an outlet for some of his frustrations through physical training—something that I copied and surpassed by a wide margin.

Compared to me, my three siblings fared remarkably well. They were spared from my father's violent outbursts. For some reason, only my mom and I were regularly beaten and harassed. As an adult I have tried to analyze this. I was probably too much like my father in many ways: rebellious, stubborn, and above all intellectually questioning. Despite all my inner uncertainties and low self-image.

In my early teens my allergies finally got better and I started to catch up to my peers in physical development. My need for psychological validation and to escape my inner trauma soon led me down a dangerous road. I got involved in petty thefts of motorcycles, burglaries, and also did some experimentation with alcohol and tobacco. In other words, I'd turned into a typical teenage inner-city thug.

I'd always done well academically at school, but when my grades plummeted into the abyss something had to be done, or I would derail completely.

The last straw was when Royal Artillery Captain Lundgren opened the envelope containing my sixth grade marks. He discovered that his incompetent son had got Fs in both order and conduct. "Enough!" he muttered.

After talking with my principal, my dad made the radical decision to send me "up north." I was going to live with my paternal grandparents in the small northern town of Nyland, on the beautiful Ångermanälven River. On a deeper level, Karl-Hugo probably understood that he had something to do with his son's situation. This was his way of killing three birds with one stone. He wouldn't have to deal with my problems. I was getting too big for him to beat up anyway. Plus I would be removed from the city suburb's dangerous environment and dark temptations. I was on my way to reform school.

In retrospect, I have to say that it was an enlightened decision on the part of my father. Of course, I didn't dare to object. I would miss my friends in Stockholm, but understood that I was on the wrong path in life. It would be a huge relief to forget the confrontations with Dad for a year or so. My trip up north would prove to last a whole lot longer than that.

Many of my friends from those years are sadly gone now. Dead from drug overdoses, accidents, or suicide.

I could have been one of them.

It requires willpower, determination, and patience to be able to change your life. Not least when it comes to changing your physique and staying in shape. Unfortunately, our current way of life demands that everything has to happen quickly. There doesn't seem to be enough time for reflection and analysis of a situation. Everything must happen at broadband speeds and we're always looking for quick fixes to all our problems. Including our health. Unfortunately, many people who want to improve their overall fitness give up too early, before any lasting results are achieved. Why? lifestyle is not something you organize over a coffee break.

I always try to remember that my health comes first. It can be a struggle to fit my training schedule into an already fully packed agenda. I work fifteen hours a day on action-movie film sets and travel across the globe most of the year. I also have to make sure that I'm there for my friends and family. Plus appear on talk shows, photo shoots, etc. Despite this, most people say that I'm in just as good or better shape today than I was twenty years ago. How do I pull that off?

After thirty-five years as an athlete and after shooting more than fifty action films, I have developed a training system that gives the best possible results over time. That's what this book is all about.

So back to how it all started: at thirteen years old I was sent away from home and became a resident of the grim northern provinces of Sweden.

Although I had spent many summer holidays with my paternal grandparents, it was a completely different matter to actually live there, go to school there, and grow up there.

I didn't have much self-confidence. Finding new friends and being respected wasn't easy. I started in my usual style: I sported long hair, smoked cigarettes, and basically gave off a bad attitude both left and right. I thought my thuggish behavior would impress everybody.

Pretty soon I discovered a huge and important difference between the northern social scene and the city I'd just come from. In the Stockholm suburbs, it was the unkempt and cocky gangster types who impressed everybody and got the hottest girls. Up north, the exact opposite was true. This was something new to me. You could safely say it was a much healthier culture.

Up north, the guys who got the most respect and were favored by the girls were the better-behaved, athletic guys. They worked out, had muscles, and were good at sports, especially ice hockey.

I soon figured out how my new environment worked. I had also become curious about the cute northern girls, so I immediately began to practice with the local hockey team. It was the first time

that I became involved in physical training in an organized manner. Off-season training in the summer consisted of sprinting up a steep muddy ski hill with the taste of blood in our mouths, then doing strength training with rusty iron bars that were stored behind the hockey rink. "Remember, fellas. When you puke, you got sixty percent left!" roared Bosse, our passionate hockey coach, in his dark blue tracksuit made of the new super-material of the day, Lycra.

Ice training started in October. I became the goalie who refused to wear a woolen cap under his plastic helmet, even when the mercury fell to a brutal ten degrees below zero. "It doesn't look good." If you want to do something right, you might as well go for it. That was a mentality I must have inherited from my over-ambitious father.

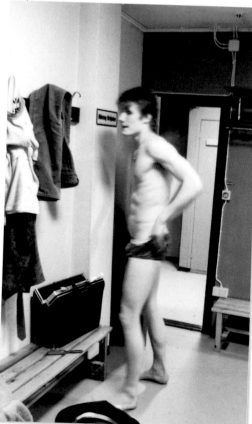

The hockey team was my gateway to serious training

18

I had also begun to grow quickly, mainly in height. To the extent that I got light-headed every time I got up from the dinner table after a hearty Swedish meal of grilled venison or black pudding. A few muscles had started to appear, possibly because of the twenty-five push-ups I rigorously churned out every night at bedtime.

Having gained some forward momentum, I decided to follow in my father's military footsteps and join both the ROTC and the Swedish Youth National Guard. We did everything from rifle target shooting to winter survival training in the snow. The worn out and fringed leather jacket that used to hang in my closet had been replaced by a green field uniform and a hockey trunk. My self-esteem was slowly returning and I realized that physical training and sports made me feel surprisingly good.

I had begun a new life.

If you're willing to accept the fact that exercise should be a part of your average day, then I have conveyed the essence of my life philosophy. Physical training that produces tangible results doesn't have to be complicated. Exercise can make you a stronger, healthier, and more complete person. The workouts that you and I will create, totaling just a few hours a week, can change the way you live your life.

AND REMEMBER: I believe in you. ○

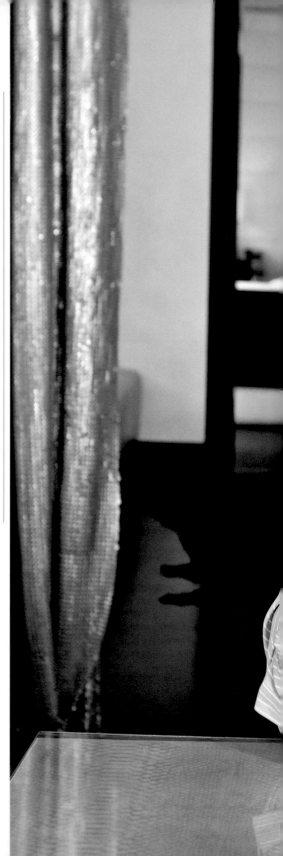

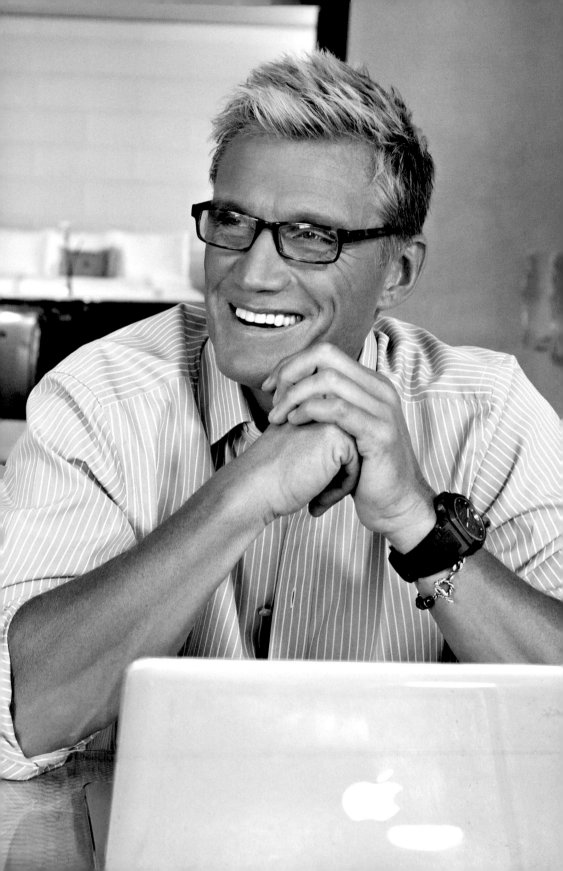

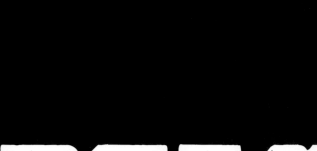

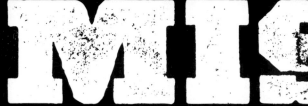

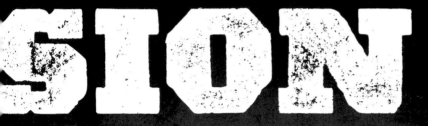

ARE YOU READY FOR THE MISSION OF YOUR LIFE?

"No pain, no gain."
With the right tools, planning and determination you will achieve your fitness goals. Are you ready?

I was in my teens, living in a small northern Swedish town. The northern babes hadn't warmed up to me yet, so it looked like I'd have to wait for that to happen.

The inner-city thug had begun to pay more attention to studying and I was also putting my best efforts into ice hockey. The local team had played in the Premier League twenty years ago and that proud memory lived on in the community. I was still a bit too thin for the contact sport and wasn't great on skates. So I got stuck as a goalie.

Ice hockey was my gateway into competitive sports and exercise. To improve my game and maybe even get picked for the nationally televised "Hockey Puck" Tournament, the dream of all northern teenagers, I needed to put on more muscle.

One of the reserve goalkeepers on the B-team was a giant named Lars, who had huge, muscular arms and wore coke-bottle eyeglasses. The occasional slap shot would miss his goaltender glove and hit him in the head. Goalies didn't wear a helmet in those days. Maybe because of those stray shots, he never seemed to have much to say. He was always lumbering around the clubhouse, mumbling to himself, while cleaning the toilets and the locker rooms. Sometimes while driving the Zamboni ice-cleaner during period breaks at A-team matches. "A damn recluse," we thought. But there was one thing he was good at: lifting barbells.

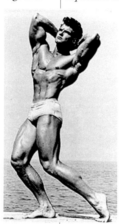

Progressive strength training with weights was a new phenomenon in the seventies. The hockey team had access to a small, ramshackle weight room, situated between the locker room and the sauna. "Big Lars" had claimed this as his domain. Woe to anyone who entered uninvited.

One day, I snuck into the weight room and snooped around. Large posters showing various weight training exercises hung on the walls. Photos of fancy American bodybuilders with slicked-back hair and bulging muscles made of steel. The greatest image of all was of Steve Reeves, one of the first celebrities of the bodybuilding world. Reeves had his heyday in the fifties, then went to Hollywood and made a career as an action star. Two decades

before anybody had heard of Arnold Schwarzenegger. In other words, he was a role model and inspiration for young Mr. Lundgren, hanging on that weight room wall.

Big Lars's exercise equipment was of serious caliber, albeit rusty and worn-out. The skinny guys on the junior team stared wide-eyed at his huge muscles bulging under a sweaty tank top. He executed lying dumbbell presses with a rusty hundred-pound dumbbell in each hand. Lars was real *superman* in our eyes.

After finishing a set he dropped the dumbbells, making the concrete floor shake. Spitting out a brownish stream of chewing tobacco he yelled at us kids, "What the hell you looking at, you bloody wimps? Get outta here!"

It was a brutal introduction to the strength training world and perhaps not entirely inspiring, but it lit a fire inside of me. Finally, I gathered some courage and asked Lars for permission to use his equipment. He reluctantly gave in and I was finally in my first gym. I immediately started to outdo myself on the bench press. When competing against my team buddies, I lost all too often. This added even more fuel to my thirst for vengeance. Every morning and night in my room, I churned out push-ups and sit-ups like crazy.

Soon, my time would come. Soon.

GET THE BODY YOU WANT

Nobody denies that a nice perk of being physically fit is a good outward appearance. Most guys want to look good both in a suit and T-shirt. We want to look in shape, our muscles clearly defined without being too huge or over the top.

Starting with the ancient Greeks, man has always strived for the ideal human physique. Statues and frescos in Athens depicted great athletes and famous warriors. The Greeks developed a system of physical training for their military units. They also created the Olympic Games. The first games are said to have taken place in the eighth century   and were held annually for a period of a thousand years. The ancient games, as do our modern Olympics, increase the society's awareness

Above: Steve Reeves
Right: A teenage Dolph in fighting stance

of exercise and physical health. Sports heavily influence our perception of the ideal human body.

When evaluating different forms of exercise, I'll watch the top athletes' bodies to determine the effect a certain sport would have on me. In engineering terms, this is called "extrapolating." You increase one variable to the extreme to get a better idea of what impact that variable has on the entire process. By studying a top athlete you'll get an idea of what physical effect that sport will have on a practitioner.

For example, a long-distance runner has a particular physique, while an elite swimmer has another. A short-distance sprinter has a third, and so on. The decathlete or boxer, who has an extremely varied training schedule, usually has a balanced and aesthetically pleasing physique.

You get the body you train for. If you want a well-balanced physique, you can't only do strength training or only run the track.

You need to vary your workouts.

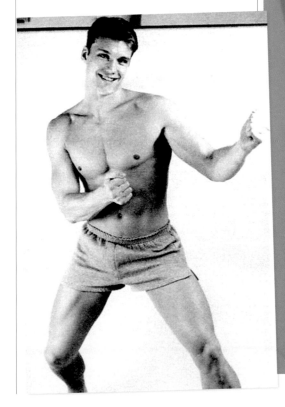

SYMMETRY AND BODY IDEAL

What goals do you have for your workout? What type of body do you want? When I started training, Steve Reeves (the bodybuilder on the ice hockey gym's wall, aka "Hercules") was my great physical ideal. Reeves is still considered to have had one of the most symmetrical bodies of all time. For me it has always been important to achieve physical symmetry.

Let's take a look at Steve Reeves's body measurements at the height of his fame.

Height: 6 feet
Weight: 216 pounds
Biceps: 18.5 inches
Calves: 18.5 inches
Neck: 18.5 inches
Thighs: 27 inches
Chest: 54 inches
Waist: 30 inches

Notice that Reeves's biceps, neck, and calves had the exact same dimensions. This is considered to be the cornerstone of physical symmetry.

Reeves's physique, transposed to various other height–weight ratios, looks like this:

5'7"–176 pounds
5'11"–203 pounds
6'3"–243 pounds

I'm 6'3", but weigh "only" 230 pounds. So, I'm a bit thin compared to Steve. On the other hand, Reeves was a bodybuilder and while I lift weights, I also practice karate, which is an endurance-based sport and results in a trimmer physique. The guy in the karate dojo who looks the slimmest can have the most dangerous and explosive knockout kick. An athlete's real power comes from the inside, not just from large muscles.

Another measurement of male body symmetry states that your chest should measure at least 10 inches more in circumference than your waist. I measure a 46-inch chest to a 34-inch waist, so that stacks up fairly well.

Why not take out the tape measure and do a quick check of your own measurements?

At sixteen, I finished school with decent grades and got admitted into the Natural Sciences program at the senior high school in Kramfors, a town about twelve miles down the river from Nyland, where I lived. My grandparents had finally started to feel proud of their former good-for-nothing grandson. To me, they had begun to feel more like my real parents.

Grandma spent ninety-five percent of her waking hours in the kitchen. My grandfather, who was a retired military officer and a former inspector at the local sawmill, could usually be found in his favorite leather armchair reading the newspaper, complaining over the stupidity of some local politician. During the spring thaw, he would get up from his chair, grab a shotgun and venture out into the backyard to engage in radical snow removal, north-country style. The large and dangerously pointed icicles that hung from the overhead drainpipes were brought down with a shotgun blast.

BAM!

Grandma didn't even flinch as she stood in the kitchen, baking cinnamon rolls.

BAM!

Another severed six-foot icicle crashed to the ground outside the kitchen window.

I never tasted cinnamon rolls better than Grandma's, either before or since. They were perfectly buttery, not too large, burnt slightly crispy at the bottom, and with extra brown sugar . . . mmm.

My start at Kramfors Senior High was tough. I considered myself a hillbilly from a small town and was hesitant to show up in a world metropolis like Kramfors in my unfashionable country wardrobe. I'd walk with my head lowered and eyes down, especially near the bus station where the coolest local kids and a few dangerous toughs hung out.

For some reason, one local girl had taken a particular liking to "The Stockholmer" (as I was called by the locals during my first few years in the north). Her older brother asked me if I wanted to try a sport called judo. I hardly knew what judo was but I gladly accepted because I saw it as a chance to see a little more of his sister.

In Sweden in the seventies, martial arts were considered mysterious and almost criminal. It seemed wrong for a real man to get involved with some sort of odd pajama wrestling. However, I started training judo with my friend in the local sports hall, practicing throws, ground fighting, and various chokeholds. There was something thrilling about facing down an opponent on the mat.

During one practice session I ended up underneath an older, overweight, and overly aggressive guy. He grabbed me in a chokehold, perspiring profusely as he bore down on my neck with loud grunts. I did everything I could to escape, but in vain. Lying there, struggling to escape from a puddle of his sweat, judo no longer felt as exciting to me.

This was not the end of martial arts in my life. Actually, it was just the beginning. Another friend, Jeff, had purchased a small book called *Karate*, written by a Hungarian former refugee, Attila Meszaros. He was one of the first practitioners of the "Kyokushinkai" style of karate in Sweden. It was a style that focused on weight training, full contact sparring, and breaking techniques— boards and bricks punched and kicked to pieces.

"Holy shit," we thought. This was something we couldn't miss!

Oddly enough, there happened to be a karate club nearby, up in the backwoods where I lived. Karate was an even more exotic and strange activity to locals than judo.

"What the hell do you think are you doing, Lundgren?" enquired my PE teacher. He had heard that of a number of lunatics dressed in white pajamas had been seen running through the snowy streets at night. Crazy maybe, but for me it was like coming home. Karate suited me perfectly, offering tougher physical exercises and greater demands for courage than judo.

Success in karate requires strength, agility, and stamina. A practitioner of karate has to be willing to embrace pain in no small measure. You'll take a beating sooner or later whether you like it or not. Besides sparring, there were stretching, push-ups, sit-ups, frog jumps, running, and other pleasantries. Cross training, we call it today. Recommended by personal trainers around the world for a well-balanced physique.

> **IT SEEMED DOWNRIGHT WRONG FOR A REAL MAN TO GET INVOLVED IN SOME SORT OF ODD PAJAMA WRESTLING.**

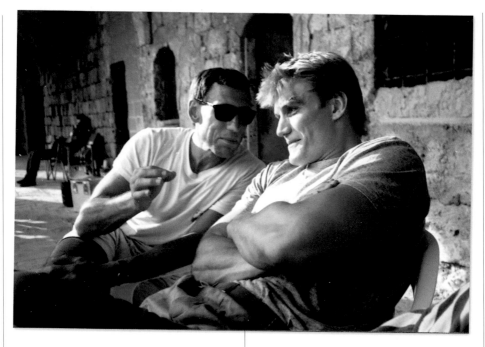

In the room next to the karate room were the weightlifters. After a year of karate, I started to throw in a little barbell training, mainly to increase my strength and improve my athletic ability. I focused on bench presses, overhead presses, and squats. These are basic strength exercises, which help you be a more effective athlete. You'll learn more about this later.

On school holidays, I took the twelve-hour train ride down to Stockholm and trained with none other than Brian Fitkin—a two-hundred-pound English karate champion who had just returned from two years of hard training in Tokyo, where he apparently had swept the floor with the Japanese fighters. Brian had won both the European and World Championships and I had so much respect for him that I started shaking as soon as he came near me during training. He was highly lethal during sparring, but at the same time had a fairness and respect for everybody in the dojo that I admired.

Shihan (Master) Brian Fitkin became my idol and father figure during those critical teenage years. We are still close friends today, having experienced many martial arts and Hollywood adventures together.

My progress in karate finally earned me some respect back up north. Pretty soon, word got around my school and to friends. "He trains karate and can break a piece of wood with one chop!"

Down in Stockholm, my dad had calmed down considerably. I had become too big and too strong to argue with, so he gave up on me. Instead, he focused on terrorizing my mother when I wasn't around. This was agonizing to me, especially since she always considered herself to be at fault. She was told daily how "she'd never be able to do anything right." Just what my dad had told me. I had escaped his sphere of influence, but she hadn't.

Many a night I lay awake in my grandparents' house, looking out the window at the greenish Northern Lights in a black sky and planned how I would beat him up. I wanted to smash his face in. I never carried it out, though, which was probably a good thing. After all, my mother was an adult who made her own choices in life. I started to realize that my parents had their own lives and I had mine.

Sometimes, when my dad was in a good mood he would say to us kids: "If you want to become some-body, you have to go to America. Over there, a man

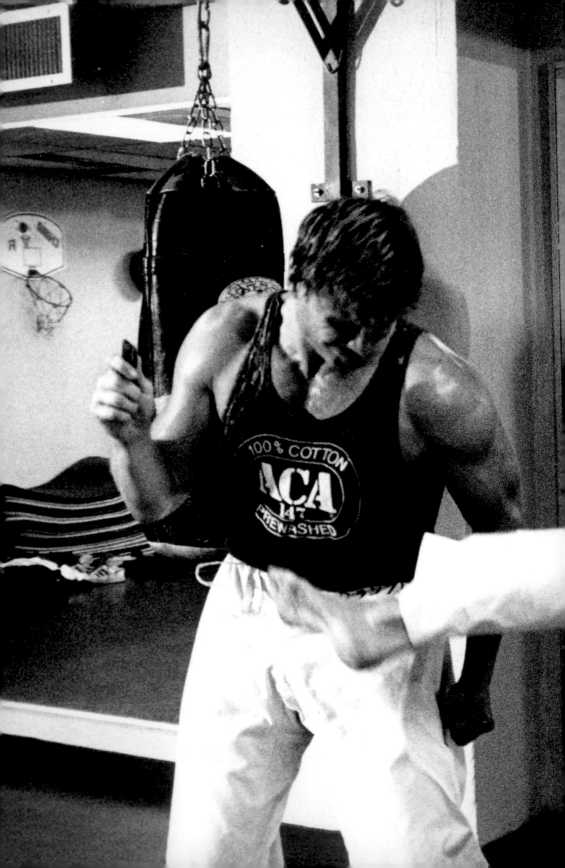

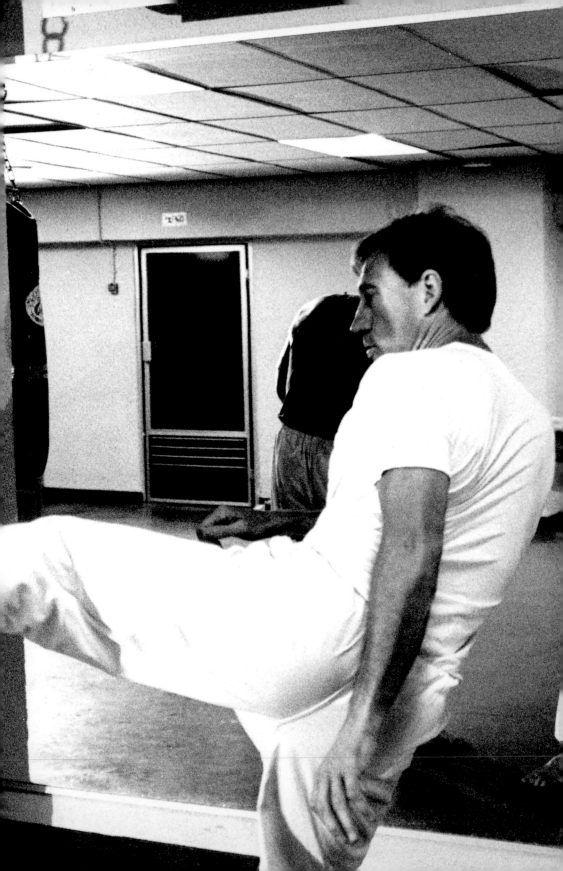

MEASURING PERFORMANCE

Now that you are committed to physical training, you need to know how your physical performance measures up. The tests described below are an easy way to check how your training pays off.

US Navy SEALs

The US Navy's famed Special Forces have a fitness test that they use to screen new recruits:

Swim 500 yards in 12.5 minutes or less, rest 2 minutes
Do at least 42 push-ups in 2 minutes, rest 2 minutes
Do at least 50 sit-ups (old-fashioned, with your heels on the floor and your hands behind your head) in 2 minutes, rest 2 minutes
Do at least 6 pull-ups (from a dead hang), rest 2 minutes
Run 1.5 miles in 12 minutes or less in marching boots

Try it! This is an indicator of true physical fitness, the kind a fighting man needs on the battlefield.

If you want to try the Navy SEAL test at the gym, skip the swimming and add 50 squats or more in 2 minutes. Make sure you bend your knees down to a 90-degree angle (use a bench or something similar to find the correct level).

As a beginner, if you are able to do 30 push-ups/sit-ups/squats in 2 minutes, that's pretty good. If you can you only do 10, you definitely need to keep reading.

1-RM

For those of us who like weight training, there's a standard test called 1-RM (One Repetition with Maximum weight)—that is, how much weight you can lift one time in various strength exercises, usually the bench press, deadlift and squat or leg press.

An excellent result is to lift your own weight in the bench press and double your body weight in the squat/leg press. In my case, this means 220 lbs and 440 lbs, respectively.

It's important to be careful with this particular test because of the risk of injury when executing a max lift. Instead, check your "10-RM" and "5-RM," that is, how much weight you can lift 10 and 5 times, respectively.

Harvard Box Test

One of the easiest fitness tests was developed for US recruits during World War II and is called the "Harvard Box Test."

In the most basic version, use a one-foot-tall box, step, or something similar. Step up with your left leg, right leg up, left leg down, right leg down. The rate should be two steps a second for 3 minutes, and check your pulse immediately afterward. A pulse rate of 80 beats per minute is a good result; higher than 120 means you need to do more cardio.

can do anything with his life. Impossible in this damn socialist country!"

I had always wanted to get out of Sweden to see the world and whether my dad was right or not, I had contracted an incurable urge to travel.

During the final years of high school, I felt the pieces of my life finally began to fall into place. For the first time ever, people actually started to look at me with respect. It was a strange and intoxicating feeling. I had been shy and withdrawn, beaten down by my dad and felt like a wimp nobody cared about. Through sports, I had finally regained much of my self-esteem.

The martial arts had found a special place in my life and had become an important part of my identity. A part that I will always carry with me.

I graduated from high school in Kramfors with a 5.0 GPA and applied for a scholarship from the Sweden–America Foundation to study in the USA. After waiting for six months I found out that I was going to Washington State University to study Chemistry. Finally in America! The year went by fast. I had to study hard for my scholarship, but there was no way I was going to take a break from training. Quite the contrary; I trained almost every day of my first year in the US. I lifted weights, boxed, and practiced the Korean martial art of Taekwondo while shaking test tubes in the university chem lab.

At the age of twenty I returned to Sweden, enrolled at the Royal Institute of Technology in Stockholm and continued to pursue my karate training. Again under the leadership of my role model Brian Fitkin at the "Stockholm Karate Kai" Club in Stockholm.

My very first sparring session back was especially memorable.

I had been practicing Taekwondo in the United States, so I was used to doing more high kicks than the others at my level. Unfortunately, I was a rookie compared to Brian. He often sparred with the students back in those days. He called me over, we bowed, and started to spar.

As he looked over to say something to another student, I delivered a kick that nailed him right in the head. His eyes flashed and he came straight back at me. A foot sweep combined with a straight punch was one of his favorite techniques and I got ready for his attack. Unfortunately he stepped in a sweat puddle, slipped, and fell hard on his back. BAM!

Everyone stopped sparring. The dojo went completely silent as the students stared first at me, then him. I stood there frozen, staring. In slow motion, I watched the European heavyweight champion get up and come at me. This time it was for real.

I never experienced such a beating in the dojo before, or since. When Brian was finished, there was a big cut under my right eye and blood trickling from my mouth from his punches. I had probably been knocked to the floor at least twenty times.

I still have a scar under one eye as a friendly reminder of that evening.

Later, Brian said he had realized something that time: there was something special about the skinny kid with the high kicks. I had never given up, no matter how many times I was knocked down. Even the great Brian Fitkin was a bit impressed.

"It's not how hard you fall; it's how quickly you get up!"

I practically lived at the karate dojo. I lifted weights and instructed beginners by day. In the evenings, I attended Brian's grueling karate sessions, sometimes twice a night.

I had developed a constant need to feel at my physical peak. It reached its most extreme when I was twenty-two years old, doing my compulsory military service as a Navy Commando in the Stockholm archipelago. During the day I crawled around in the trenches carrying an assault rifle, paddled kayaks, and ran combat assault courses with my enlisted buddies. In the evening I took the ferry from the island where I was stationed, catching the bus to Stockholm for a hard karate workout. I came back home again by bus and ferry, entering the barracks at 11:30 p.m. to hang up my wet karate uniform, when the others were already snoring in their beds. The reveille at 5:30 a.m. for another day's work always came too soon.

Looking back, I'd become a true fitness fanatic. But this was how I found the focus and discipline that was to prove useful later in life. I felt as if no physical challenge was too tough, that anything was possible once I decided to do it.

After finishing my military service, I went back to the Royal Institute of Technology. Later that year, I took my black belt in "Kyokushinkai" karate. At the time of my black belt grading, I had applied for a scholarship to study Chemical Engineering at Sydney University in Australia. I was awarded the scholarship and was off to Australia for a full year.

My dad drove me down to the station to take the commuter train to Stockholm, then the shuttle bus to the airport. Mom rode next to him. In the trunk sat one very large and heavy suitcase. Not enough for a whole year, but it was all they would allow me to bring on my low-price economy ticket.

I noticed that my father became very emotional when he shook my hand to say goodbye. In that moment, I suddenly felt that the past was now forgotten and only the future mattered.

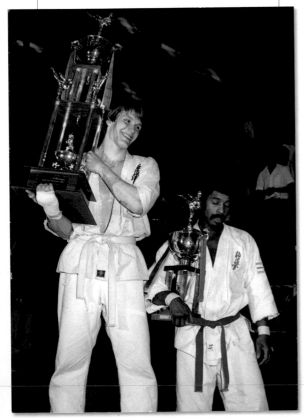

Winner of the British Open Knockdown Karate Tournament 1980

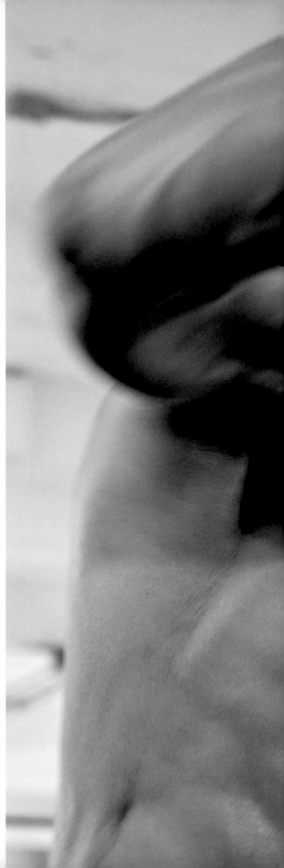

Through the train window, I watched the image of my parents standing on the station platform slowly disappearing from view. I sat back in the vinyl seat and took a deep breath: I was finally on my way.

FULLY INTEGRATED TRAINING—"FIT"

When it comes to scheduling physical training, you can't ignore the other aspects that shape your daily life. My training system is designed to work anytime, even on a very busy schedule.

Like most of us, I have a life full of obligations: a demanding job, a family to care for, travel, and so on. I find myself always on the move, sometimes more than two hundred days in a year. That's why I have focused on high intensity training and a combination of different exercises that keep your body guessing. I use workout routines that ensure a good training effect and fit into a hectic daily schedule. My "FIT," a "Fully Integrated Training" system is flexible and designed to fit the demands of everyday life.

Because of my job, it's very difficult to plan ahead. However, I always try to schedule the upcoming week. How many workouts I can get in and what they will consist of.

Sometimes I have a bigger objective: "I have to be in top shape for a movie in two months." Or, "I feel I'm losing some cardio. I have to do more of that." I'll adjust the workouts accordingly with a focus on the special training that brings me closer to my target.

I've learned not to be a time-optimist, but rather to be a bit critical of my initial plans, "Do I really have time to squeeze in those four strength sessions at the gym during this busy week?" If it seems like it will be difficult to find the time, I'll replace some of the longer sessions with the No Excuses home fitness workouts you'll read about later. In these instances, I'll usually train in the mornings before breakfast, when I have the most control over my time.

This book contains no workout "secrets," no "magic" exercises, or "revolutionary" equipment. If you have had any previous experience in strength training you will probably recognize most of what I'm talking about. It's in the combination of the different exercises that the great benefit will be found. It's how you plan your weekly and monthly schedules that give you the edge.

Getting in great shape requires hard work. You know it and I know it. There are no short cuts. But there is a smart way to do it. ○

Okay, enough talking.

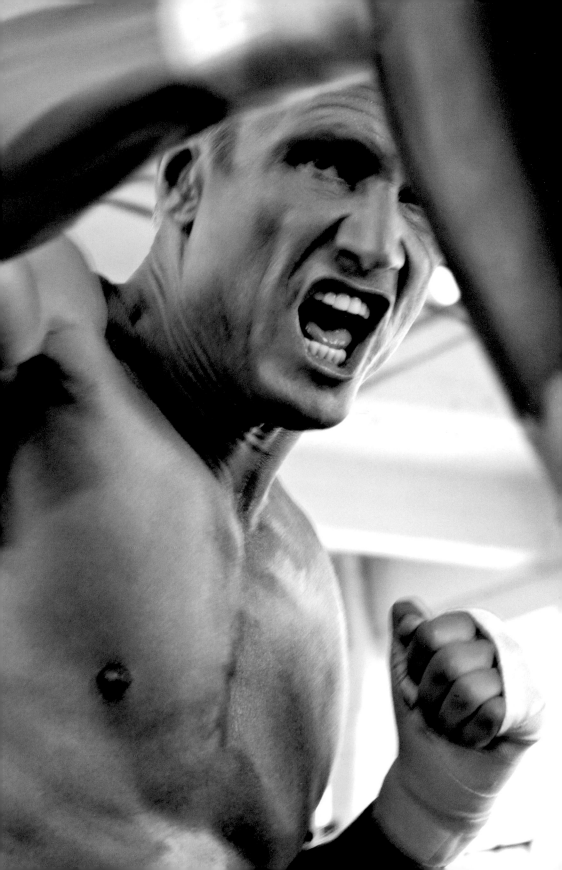

Self defense in the street is not like in the movies. Or in the ring. Things happen very quickly and violently. There are no second chances. The only way to escape somebody who's trying to hurt you is for you to hurt them more. That's the brutal truth.

Practice these moves carefully with a partner and you'll feel more confident. Ready to handle yourself in the unlikely event of an attack. The more you practice, the better you'll get.

NSE SYSTEM

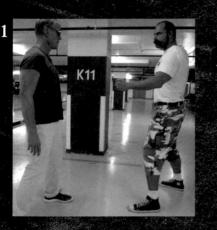

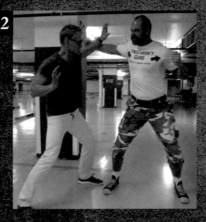

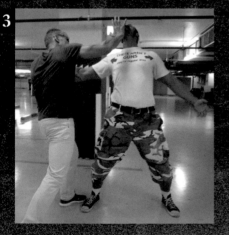

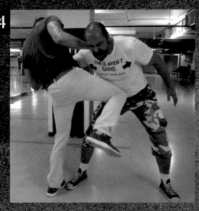

AGAINST A RIGHT PUNCH

Step in and block using your forearm [2].
Use a palm heel strike to the chin or the nose. Better than a punch and easier to hit the target [3].
Follow up with a knee strike to the groin [4].

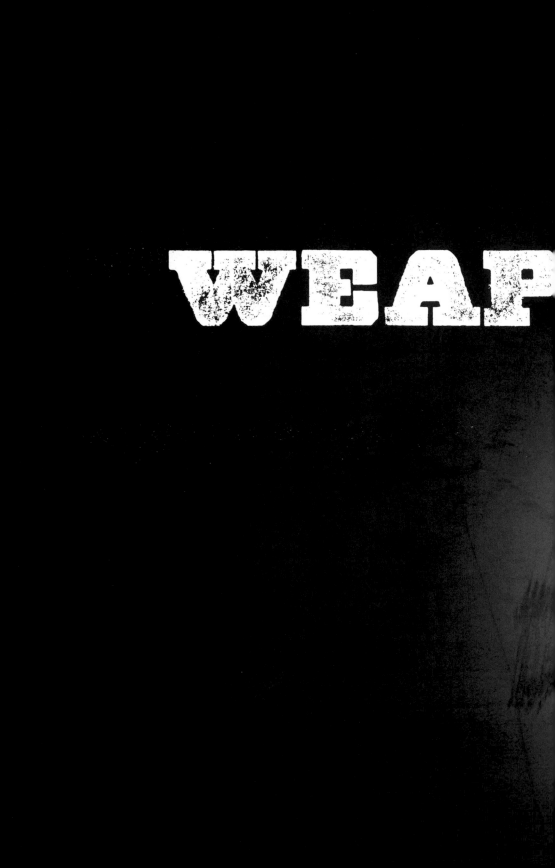

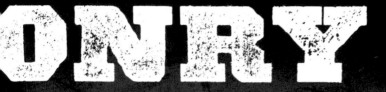

YOUR EXERCISE ARSENAL AND HOW TO USE IT

Over the past thirty years, I've pushed my way through thousands of workouts, trying and evaluating most of the training regimes out there.

Through blood, sweat, and tears, I developed my own training system that is hard to beat in terms of versatility, adaptability, and results.

Now you too can benefit from this experience.

DL'S FIT TRAINING SYSTEM "FULLY INTEGRATED TRAINING"

The most important factor for staying fit is variety. Through variety, you can ensure that your entire body gets what it needs. Once you create a solid foundation, you'll be well equipped to achieve lasting results.

You can build on this foundation for the rest of your life.

MY THREE PARTS OF PHYSICAL FITNESS

A training schedule must be simple. Ideally, a number of basic training programs that you combine with each other, depending on your fitness goals and how much time you have.

I split my training into three main parts:
1. **Strength training**
2. **Endurance training**
3. **Stretching and flexibility training**

I usually combine these parts to fit my current needs. It is easy for you to do the same.

1. Strength training includes a variety of exercises with weights.

2. Endurance training includes boxing, karate, swimming, running, and other activities that enhance endurance, coordination, and your aerobic capacity.

3. Stretching and flexibility includes stretching, relaxation, and meditation.

In Chapter 4, Special Ops, I cover a number of special workout programs. This covers training at home and routines that you can use when you're traveling.

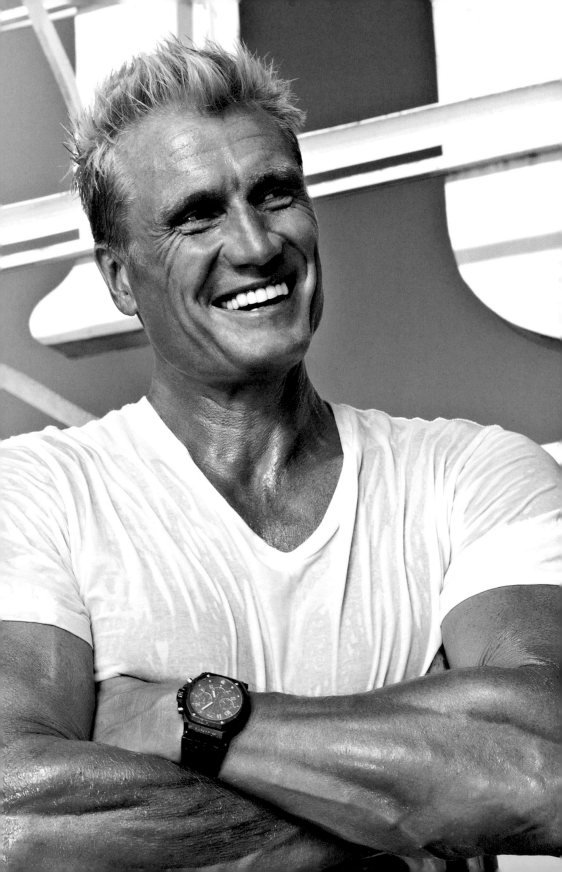

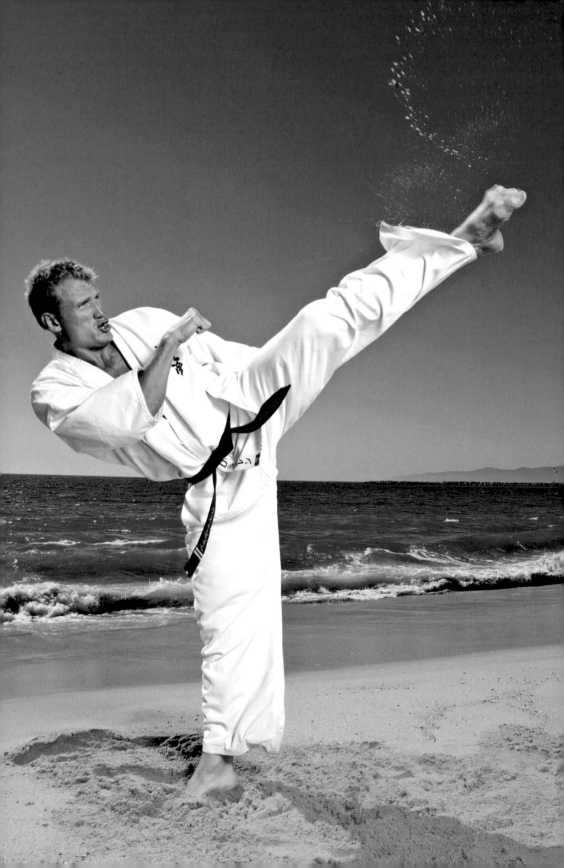

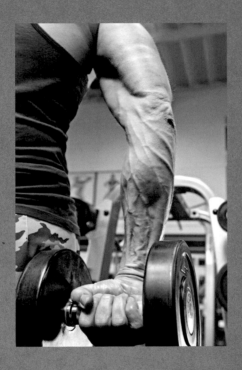

STRENGTH TRAINING

I have always used weight training to stay fit, especially when preparing for different film roles. Sure, you can get good results through callisthenic exercises like push-ups and sit-ups, but to effectively build muscle mass you need to train with weights.

Weight training strengthens your joints and ligaments and improves your muscular power. For all athletes, weight training is essential to improve performance and to prevent injuries.

The older you get, the more important strength training becomes. Genetically speaking, humans lose about ten percent of muscle mass every ten years after reaching middle age. To curb this negative trend and maintain muscle mass, you need strength training.

Muscles are extremely energy consuming, so the more muscle mass you have, the more fat you will burn, even when you're not exercising.

Weight training makes you stronger and more muscular, reduces body fat, and prevents aging. What are you waiting for?

MACHINES VERSUS FREE WEIGHTS

A weight machine's positions and trajectories are fixed, which helps you perform the movement correctly. It also makes it harder to strain a muscle, which can happen if you use free weights incorrectly. Training with machines, however, does not provide results as quickly as using free weights.

Free weights challenge the body's core and develop muscles in a more effective manner than machines. I prefer using free weights, but for certain muscles, machine exercises are effective.

Machines work particularly well in circuit training, where you have to move quickly between workout stations. With machines, you don't waste time taking weight plates on and off.

Machines are also very practical for injury rehabilitation. This is how many weight machines were invented.

Sometimes it can be difficult to find proper free weights, especially in places like a hotel gym, so I've worked some weight machine exercises into my strength training programs.

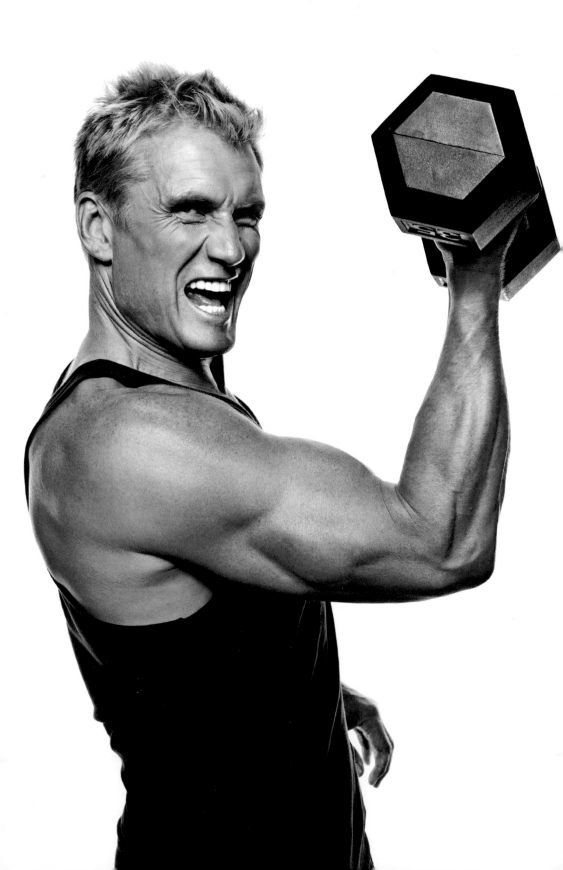

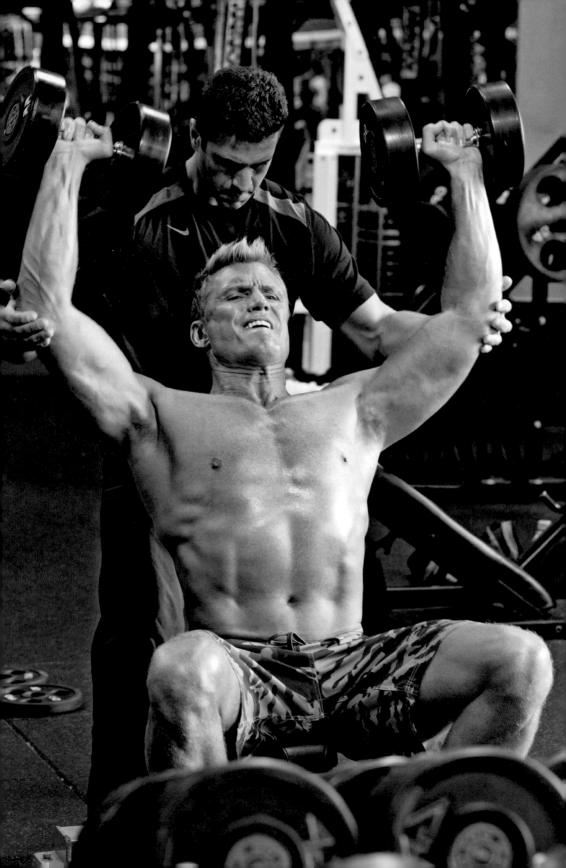

**"PUSH AND PULL ROUTINES"
—BUILD MUSCLE**

EXERCISES AND PROGRAMS

The first three programs in my system are "split" routines. The muscles of your body are divided up then exercised during three different training sessions a week. When combined, **DL Programs 1, 2**, and **3** train the entire body. Dividing up the workout, you ensure that each major muscle group gets at least forty-eight hours of rest.

DL Programs 1 and 2 are based on the "Push and Pull" principle: One day, you do "push" exercises like squats and bench presses and the next day "pull" exercises like deadlifts and lat pulls. DL Program 3 takes care of your shoulders and arms.

DL Programs 1 and 2 are the base for strength training routines used by athletes to build strength and power. Movements like squats, bench press, and deadlifts are particularly suitable if you want to increase muscle mass and strengthen your "core," i.e. the body's stabilizing muscles.

If you miss Program 3 one week, it's not the end of the world. Shoulders and arms still get some good training in the other two programs.

DL Program 4 is a special weight circuit workout to be used as a complement to the other three programs. During one circuit training session, you train the whole body using less weight but at a higher intensity. It's also aerobically challenging, because there is no rest between exercises. This type of circuit training is often used by boxers and MMA fighters when they prepare for an event.

If you only have time for one workout a week, you should do DL Program 4, because it offers a challenge for both your muscles and your cardiovascular system.

DL PROGRAM 1—OUTLINE

Warm Up (5 minutes)

Abdominals
Hanging leg lifts (3 x 15–20), 46

Lower back
Back lifts (3 x 20), 48

Front Thighs
Leg Extension (12/15/10), 48
Squats or leg press machine (15/12/8/6), 51
Leg Press—one leg at a time (15 reps per leg), 51

Chest
Bench press (15/12/8/6), 52
Dumbbell flyes or cable flyes (2 x 12), 52

Core
Ball planks/hip rotations with medicine ball
(3 supersets of 45 seconds plank on the balance ball, 30
seconds rest, 45 seconds seated hip rotations with medicine
ball—rest 30 seconds between sets), 54

DL Stretch (3 minutes)

Cardio (3 minutes)

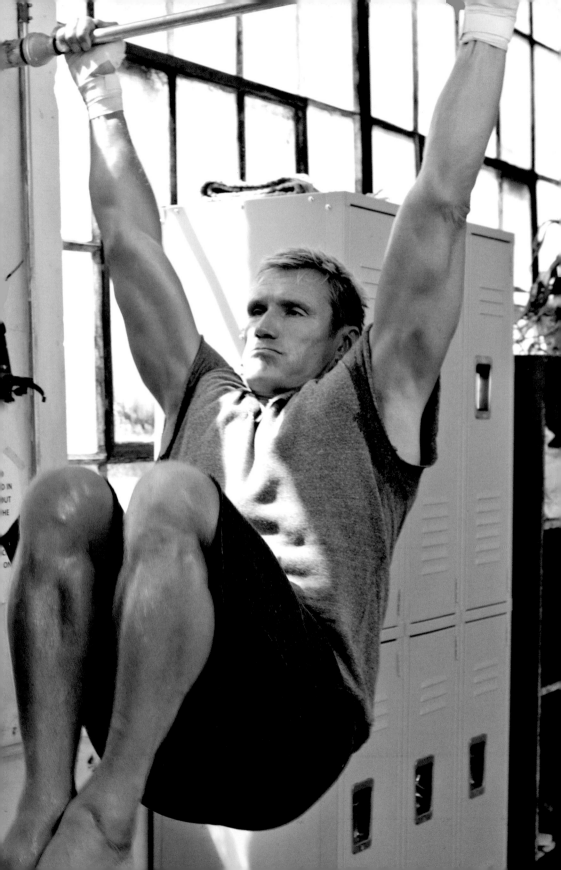

WARM UP

Five minutes on an exercise bike. Try increasing the resistance one level every minute.

This is my most common warm up, but you can use any cardio machine or run on a treadmill. Don't run too hard. This is a strength workout and we want to concentrate on the fast muscle fibers, not the slow endurance fibers used in running.

You can also do the "box test" to warm up (see Chapter 2), which is three minutes step-up and step-down on a 20-inch tall box or a bench. This is a seemingly simple exercise, but it trains both knees and your aerobic endurance in a highly effective way.

ABDOMINALS
Hanging leg lifts

Starting position: Grip a pull-up bar, or a well-secured overhead grip. The most important thing is that your legs hang freely [A1].
Execution: Tighten your abdominal muscles, raising your straight legs up in front of you. Continue until they are parallel to the floor. As you get stronger, you can take them all the way up to your head [A2]. Return, controlled, to the starting position.

You can vary this by raising your legs to the side with your knees bent, alternating sides [A3], or going out into a split [A4]. The important thing is that you feel your abdominals contracting.

I like to do hanging abdominal exercises at the beginning of a training session. It gives quick results and it also engages the forearms. Hanging exercises are very effective—just look at the amazing body of a competitive gymnast!

Try not to swing too much. This is a controlled exercise. If you have to, put your foot down on the floor to stabilize your body then keep going to finish the set. Keep your knees together throughout the leg lifts.

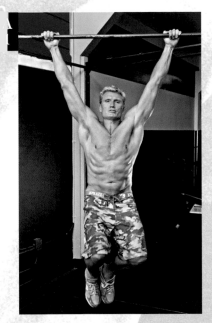

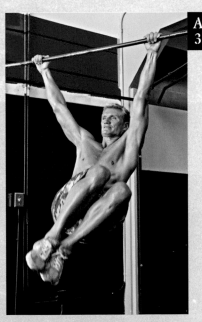

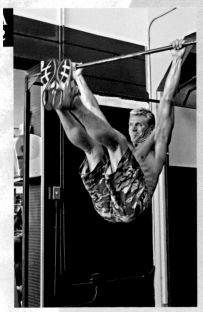

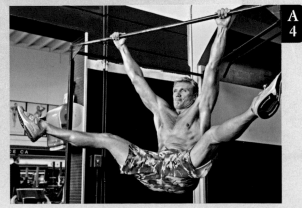

LOWER BACK
Back lift

Starting Position: Position yourself in the hyper-extension machine with your feet hip-width apart, knees slightly bent and hips against the cushion. Tighten your stomach and lower back. [A1]

Execution: "Roll" your body up until your hamstrings and back are in line with one another [A2]. It's important that you don't go too high. Return to the starting position, using a controlled movement.

As you get stronger, you can hold a weight against your chest to increase the effect [A3]. Always do the first set without added weight to warm up your back muscles.

The lumbar region is a problem area for many people, especially for those who make a living sitting down at a desk or in front of a computer. Stress, both emotional and physical, tends to manifest itself in the lumbar region, so it's important not to skip this part of your workouts.

A weak lower back will hinder you when doing other exercises. I have had a lot of problems with this, because of all the high kicks I've done in karate over the years. Back lifts have, more or less, eliminated my problem.

FRONT THIGHS
Leg extension

Starting Position: Sit on a leg extension machine with your feet hip-width apart and your knees just off the cushion. Let the cushion rest against your shins.

Execution: Using your thigh muscles, raise the cushion until your legs are fully extended [B1]. Return, controlled, to the starting position.

This exercise strengthens the muscles around your knees and also serves as a warm up for the heavier squats. Make sure you are going at a fairly slow pace and hold for a beat in the top position for maximum effect on the muscles and ligaments.

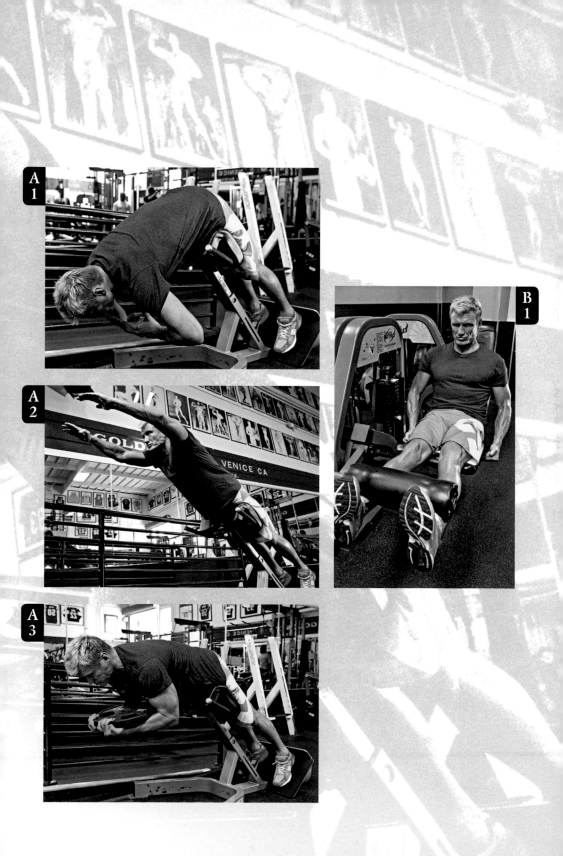

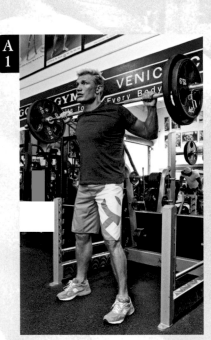

A1

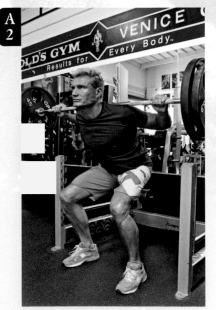

A2

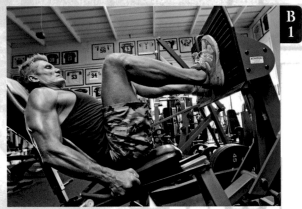

B1

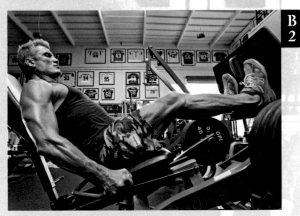

B2

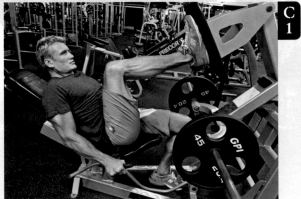

C1

FRONT THIGHS
Squats or leg press machine
Here is an exercise that hits the entire body. Squats with a barbell are preferable, but the leg press machine works too. This is truly a phenomenal strength exercise for the whole body. The guys at Gold's Gym will tell you: "If you want big biceps, do squats!"

With every set, I increase the weight and decrease the number of repetitions to increase testosterone levels and to stimulate muscle growth throughout the body. This is called doing a "pyramid"—fewer reps and more weight with each increasing set.

Squats
Starting Position: Make sure the bar is located comfortably on your shoulders. Stand with your feet hip-width apart and your knees slightly bent. Tighten your abs [A1].
Execution: Bend your knees and slowly squat down until your thighs are almost parallel to the floor [A2]. Return, controlled, to the starting position.

When you do squats, remember to start relatively light to warm up the knees and muscles. Keep your gaze directed upwards to help keep your lower back straight, which strengthens the entire lift. You should never let your thighs drop past the horizontal position. This can be harmful to the knee joint.

Squats are one of the best all-around exercises you can do and one of the "Basic Five" classic strength training exercises. The others are bench press, military press, deadlift, and rowing.

Leg press machine
Starting Position: Sit down and center yourself on the leg press machine. Make sure your feet are hip-width apart and placed firmly against the footplate [B1].
Execution: Using the entire bottom of your feet, push the plate until your legs are almost straight [B2]. Return, controlled, to the starting position.

Leg press—one at a time
We all have a certain asymmetry in our bodies, especially in the legs and hips. Normally, one leg is stronger than the other. Asymmetric training helps to strengthen the opposite sides of the body separately. Try using the leg press machine with one leg only [C1].

Use the resting leg to balance your body. Start off by choosing a light weight. This exercise is more about balance and symmetry than brute strength.

CHEST
Bench press
Starting Position: Lie on the bench with your feet on the floor. Grasp the bar with a grip that is slightly wider than shoulder width. Tighten your abs [A1].
Execution: Lower the bar to your upper chest. When the bar touches your chest, press it back up to its original position [A2].

As with squats, it is important that you start light and increase the weight as you go. Make sure not to bounce the bar off your chest, but keep good form. When using really heavy weights (i.e., more than your own bodyweight) you should have a partner to spot you.
   The bench press is one of the absolute best all-round exercises for your upper body. It's one of the "Basic Five" exercises of strength training.

Dumbbell flyes or Cable flyes
We follow up the bench press with a lighter exercise to increase the blood flow and create better muscle definition.

Dumbbell flyes
Starting Position: Grip a dumbbell in each hand. Lie on a bench with your feet firmly on the floor. Your hands should be above your head with your palms turned toward each other [B1].
Execution: In a controlled motion, lower your arms outward and downward until they are parallel to the floor (or slightly below) [B2]. Return to the starting position. Keep your arms slightly bent to take some pressure off the elbow joint.

Cable flyes
Starting Position: Connect the pulley handles to the upper cables of a two-stack cable machine. Grip the handles and lean slightly forward, standing just in front of the machine. Keep your arms slightly bent. Tighten your abs [C1].
Execution: Pull the handles down in an arc until your hands meet in front of your navel. Tighten your chest muscles for a beat [C2]. Return, controlled, to the starting position.

After doing a heavy barbell exercise, I like to use a lighter complementary exercise to focus specifically on that muscle group. Most strength programs in the book are structured in this way.

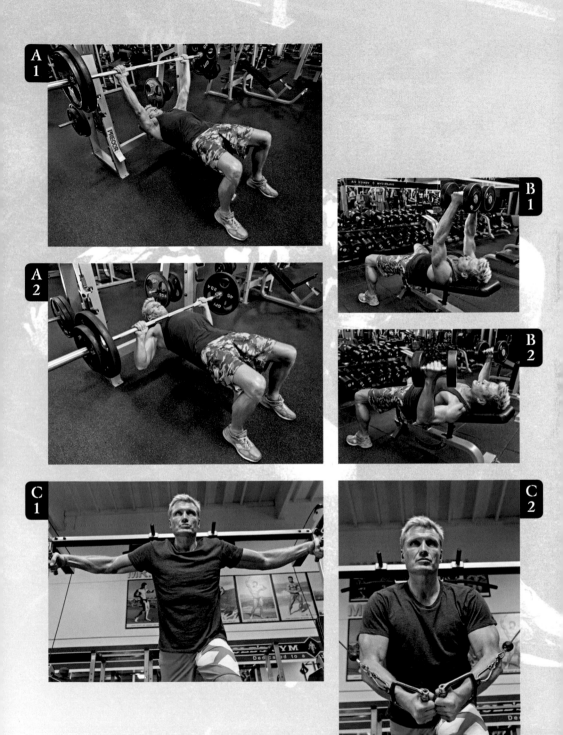

CORE
Swiss ball planks/hip rotations with medicine ball
We end the session with a core exercise. I like a combination of planks and hip rotations.

Swiss ball planks
Starting position: Place your elbows on the ball. Tighten your stomach and raise yourself up until your body is straight as a plank [A1].
Execution: Hold your body in this position for 45 seconds.

Hip rotations with medicine ball
Starting position: Sit on the floor with a medicine ball in your hands. Lift your feet off the floor with your knees slightly bent. Tighten your abs [B1].
Execution: Rotate the ball in front of your body, from side to side [B2]. Keep this up for 45 seconds.

This is a combined exercise that not only works well on the visible abdominal muscles, but also on your core, i.e., the smaller stabilizing muscles of the lower back and the deep abdominal muscles.

To further increase the effect of the Swiss ball plank you can roll the ball using your elbows, first clockwise then counterclockwise for 45 seconds [A2]. For better effect with the medicine ball rotations, bring the ball all the way down to the ground at the end of each rotation.

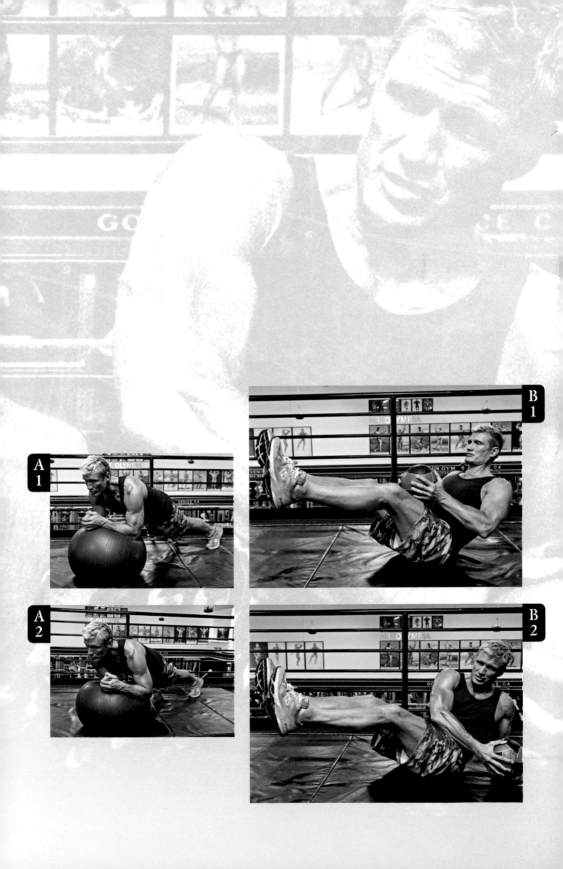

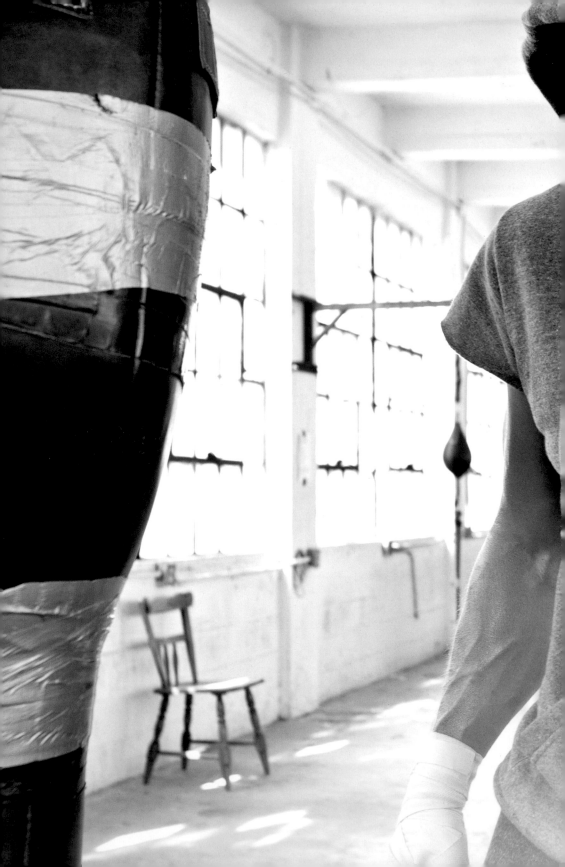

STRETCH

DL stretch (see page 110) is a short stretching program that I use after each strength workout to prevent muscle stiffness and soreness. Hold each position for 10 seconds.

LIGHT CARDIO (SHADOWBOXING, PUNCHING BAG, RUNNING, CYCLING, OR SWIMMING)

Some light cardio to wind down and relax the muscles and joints. Shadowboxing, jumping jacks, jogging, or similar activities work well to prevent soreness and speed up recovery. If you have a pool in your gym, you can swim 200 meters. It's important not to do too much cardio here—we're in the gym to build muscle.

Total time for DL Program 1:60 minutes

DL PROGRAM 2— "PULL"

DL PROGRAM 2—OUTLINE

Warm up (5 minutes)

Lower back/Abdominals
Back lifts and v-ups/elbow-to-knees
(3 supersets of 20 reps per exercise), 61

Hamstrings and buttocks
Deadlifts (15/12/8/6), 62

Hamstrings
Leg curls (15/12/10), 62

Calves
Calf raises (3 x 20), 64

Forearms
Forearm curls (20/15/15: behind the back,
regular curls, reverse curls), 66

Back
Lat pull-down machine (15/12/8/6), 68
Seated row machine (2 x 12), 68
Dumbbell pullovers (15), 68

DL Stretch (3 minutes)

Cardio (3 minutes)

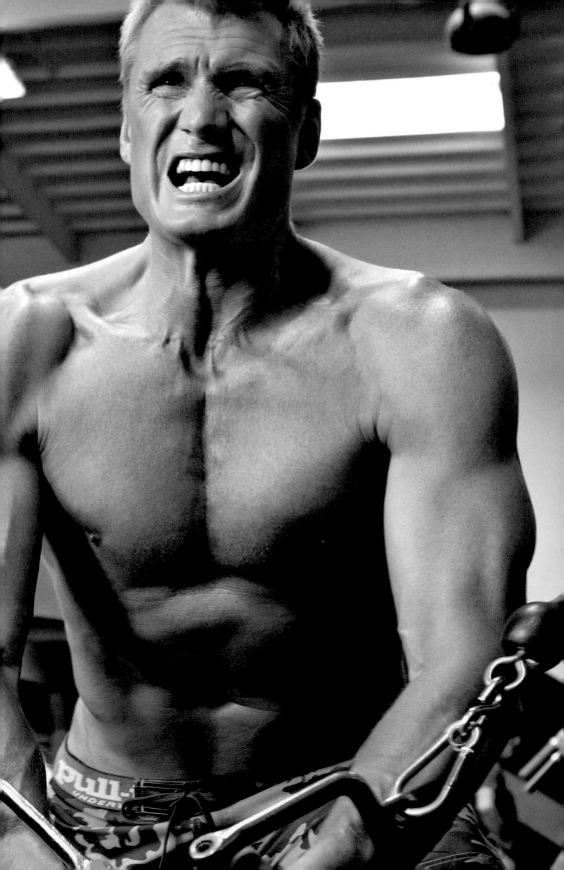

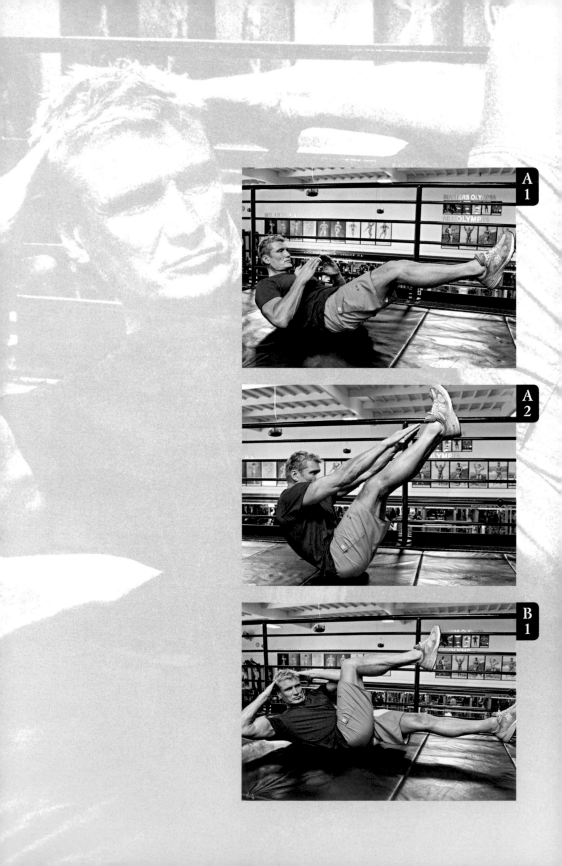

WARM UP

Warm up on the exercise bike, rowing machine or treadmill. Start easy and increase the resistance slightly as you go.

LOWER BACK/ABDOMINALS
Back lifts and v-ups/elbow-to-knees
Back lifts
See page 48.

V-ups
Starting position: Lie on the floor with your body completely straight and lift your hands and feet off the ground. Tighten your stomach, keeping your legs 4 inches above the floor [A1].
Execution: Using your abdominal muscles, raise your legs and upper body upwards [A2]. Your hands and feet should meet in the top "V" position before returning to the starting position.

Elbow-to-knees
Starting position: Lie on your back with your legs in the air. Lift your shoulders off the floor, and place your hands on either side of your head. Tighten your abs.
Execution: Use your abdominal muscles to rotate your upper body to one side while bending your leg in front of you [B1]. Bring your elbow to meet the opposite knee before returning back to the starting position. Repeat on the other side.

Try a superset of 20 back lifts with the first abdominal exercise (20 v-ups) and then rest for a minute. Then do another superset of 20 back lifts with the second abdominal exercise (20 elbow-to-knees) before you rest a minute. Do three of these supersets.

HAMSTRINGS AND GLUTES
Deadlifts
Starting position: Grip the bar with a shoulder-width grip and with your feet hip-width apart. Hold one hand with the palm facing forward and the other with the palm directed backward [B1]
Execution: While looking ahead, lift the barbell by using your legs and buttocks until your body is completely straight, keeping your eyes looking forward [A2]. Lower the bar slowly to the floor and repeat. Make sure to bend at the knees, slowly lowering the bar down on the floor, keeping your back straight and chest out. This should be a very controlled movement.

The deadlift is another one of the "Basic Five" strength training exercises. It is extremely effective, not just for the back, thighs, and buttocks, but for the whole body. Deadlifts build your core and result in a rapid increase in strength. The movement stimulates all major muscle groups and testosterone levels.

As with the all heavy lifting exercises, start easy and gradually increase the weight as your body warms up.

HAMSTRINGS
Leg curl
Starting position: Lie on your stomach on a leg curl machine. Your knees should be outside the edge of the bench and the cushioned pad should rest against the lower part of the calf muscle. Tighten your abs.
Execution: Bend your knees and, using your hamstrings, pull your heels toward your buttocks [B1]. Return, controlled, to the starting position.

Make sure you pull the weight at a steady pace, with a slight pause at both the top and bottom positions. There are also leg curl machines where you perform the same movement sitting up.

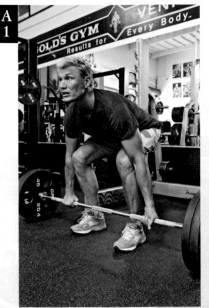

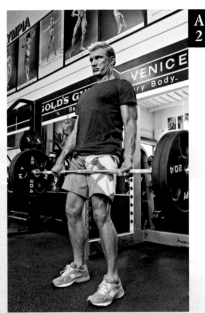

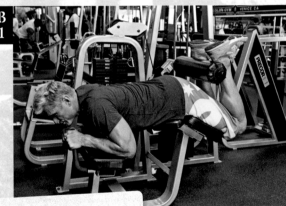

It's easy to neglect your body's "dark side," i.e. your back, hamstrings, and calves. Even though you don't see them, they are very important for the body's stability. If they are underdeveloped, you risk developing back and knee problems.

CALVES
Calf raises

Starting position: Sit on a calf raise machine. The ball of the foot should be on the step. The lever cushion should be just above the knees. Sit up straight and tighten your abs.

Execution: Raise the heel as far as you can [A1]. Stay in the top position for a beat, then return, controlled, to the starting position. Stretch the calf in the bottom position [A2]. Repeat.

This exercise can also be done in a standing calf machine.

Calves are extremely difficult to train. Most of us take around five thousand steps a day just getting around. We do thousands of calf repetitions without even visiting the gym. To give your calves more of a challenge, try doing one set with your toes straight ahead [A3], one with your toes out [A4], one with your toes inward [A5], and one more set straight ahead [A3]. This way, you work every angle of the calf muscle.

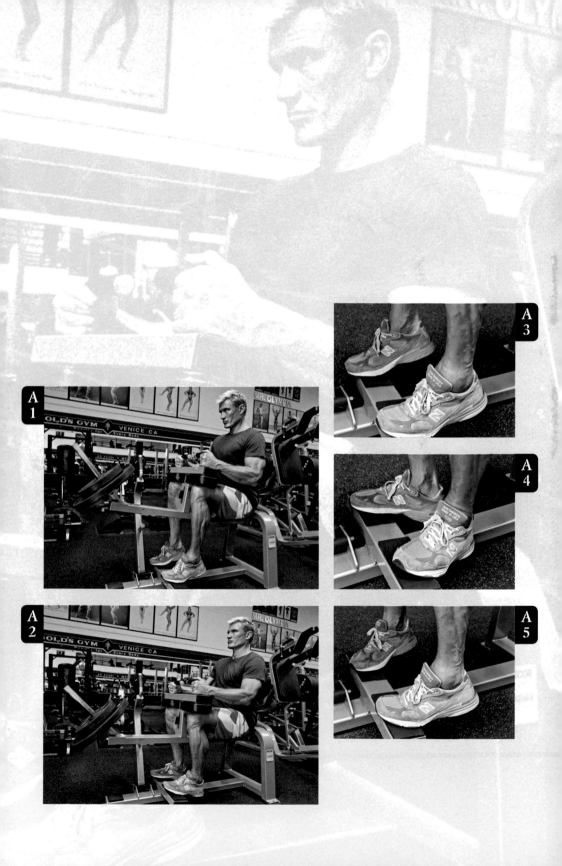

FOREARMS
Forearm curls

Starting position: Sit on a bench, holding a barbell with an underhand grip, resting your forearms on your thighs. Roll the bar down and away from you, opening your hands slightly so that the bar reaches your fingers [A1].
Execution: Curl the bar by bending first your fingers and then your hands toward you [A2]. Return, controlled, to the starting position.

This exercise can also be done with an overhand grip, in which case you should lessen the load. You can also do forearm curls standing up, curling a barbell or two dumbbells [A3] behind your back. The principle is the same.

Forearms are quite visible, when you wear a T-shirt or a shirt with rolled up sleeves. Well-trained forearms are a sure sign that a guy is fit. They happen to be my *Expendables* buddy Sly Stallone's favorite muscle group. Many men tend to neglect them, but let's face it: big upper arms and tiny forearms don't really look that great together!

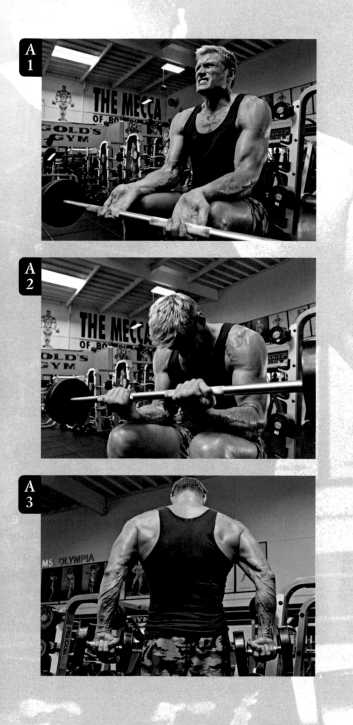

BACK

Lat pull machine

Let's start our back workout with the lat pull machine, an exercise that increases both the width and thickness of the back muscles.

Starting position: Attach a wide bar to a lat pull-down machine. Grasp the bar with a grip slightly wider than shoulder width. Sit with your feet together and your knees bent at a ninety-degree angle. Tighten you abs [A1].
Execution: Pull the bar down toward the center of your chest. Not too low or you won't get the full effect on your upper back [A2]. Inhale in the top position and exhale in the bottom position. Remember to pause for a beat in the top position to stretch out your back.

Seated row machine

Starting position: Attach a bar or handles to a rowing machine. Grip the bar. Sit with your feet hip-width apart and your knees slightly bent [B1].
Execution: Lean forward, extending your arms completely and then, first using your back muscles and then your arms, pull the bar to your stomach [B2]. Hold the end position for a beat before returning to the starting position. Repeat.

This exercise builds up the lower back and the middle of the back, closer to the spine.

You can use both the lat-pull and rowing machines with a narrow v-handle instead of a straight bar.

Dumbbell pullovers

After all the back exercises, it's time to stretch out the spine and upper body muscles properly. Try this classic body building exercise.

Starting position: Lie across a horizontal bench and hold a medium-weight dumbbell in both hands with your arms straight above your head [C1].
Execution: Inhale and lower the dumbbell backward, over your head, at the same time lowering your hips to get the maximum stretch [C2]. Then breathe out and lift the dumbbell back to the starting position. Repeat.

This exercise is said to increase your chest circumference and reportedly was one of Arnold Schwarzenegger's favorites during his Mr. Universe days.

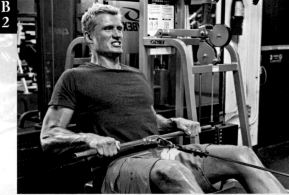
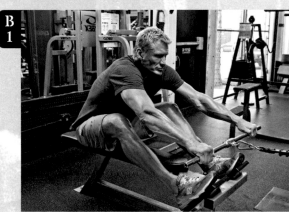
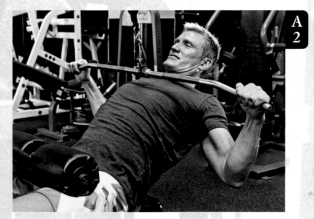
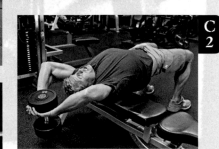

STRETCH
DL stretch (see page 110).

CARDIO
Try running, skipping rope, a punching bag, shadowboxing, cycling, or swimming.
This helps to cool down and speed up your recovery.

Total time for DL Program 2: 60 minutes

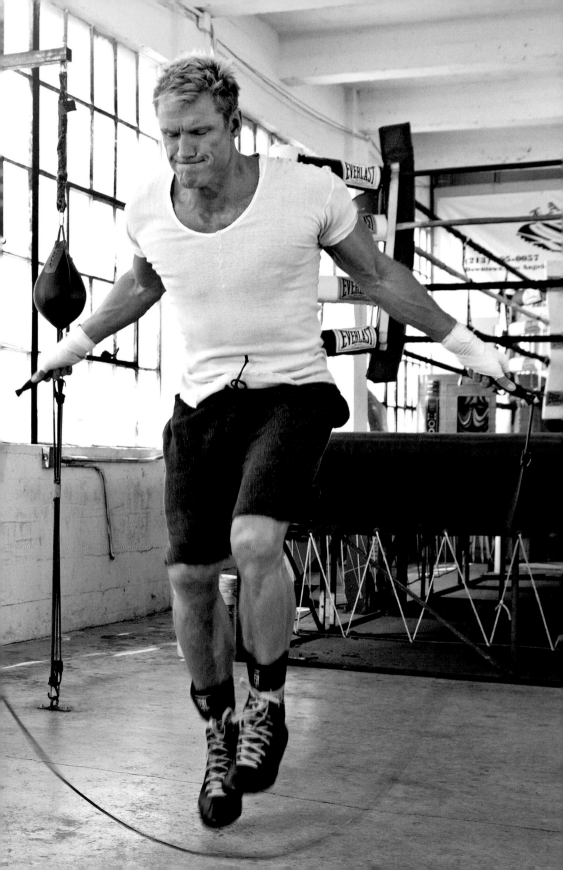

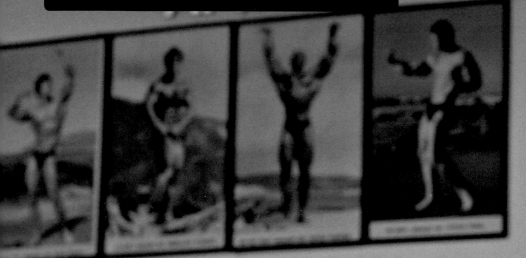

DL PROGRAM 3—"THE GUN SHOW"

This program focuses on your shoulders and arms. It's a faster and lighter workout than the two previous programs. DL Programs 1 and 2 exercise the entire body with a focus on strength and muscle mass growth. DL Program 3 is about shoulders and arms, muscles that are especially visible when you wear a T-shirt. Well-proportioned, strong arms give that masculine feel and athletic look that all men are after. Sorry, being an action star with scrawny arms just does not work. They require some special attention.

To get really impressive shoulders and arms, this session is a must!

DL PROGRAM 3— OUTLINE

Warm Up (5 minutes)

Abdominals
Hanging leg lifts (3 x 15-20),75

Shoulders
"Arnold" dumbbell press (15/12/10/8), 75
Combination exercises for shoulders (3 x 12), 75

Biceps
Standing bicep curls with dumbbells (15/12/10/8), 76
Concentration curls (2 x 15), 76

Triceps
Lying triceps press (15/12/10/8), 76
Triceps press on cable machine (2 x 15), 76

Lower back/Abdominals
Back lift/sit-ups on the ball (20 resp. 30), 78

DL stretch (3 minutes)

Cardio (3 minutes)

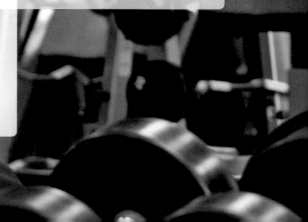

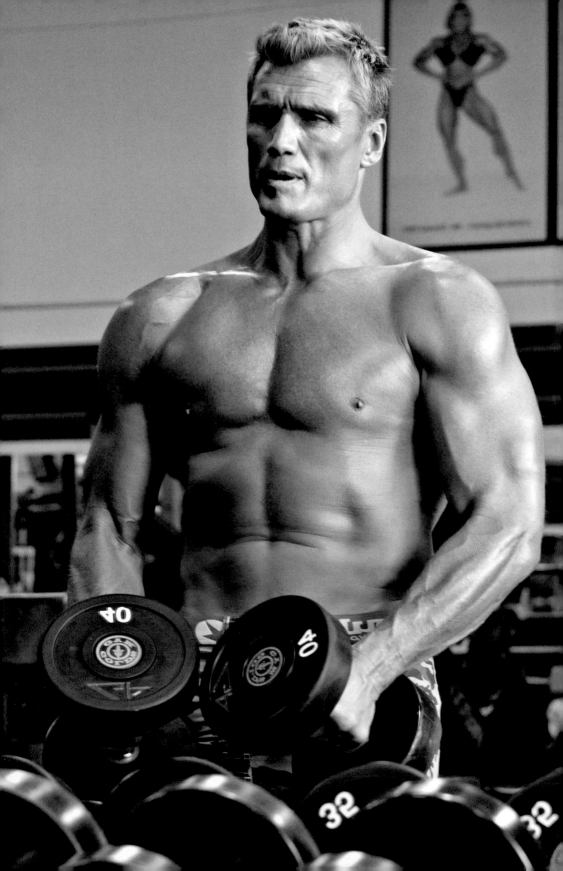

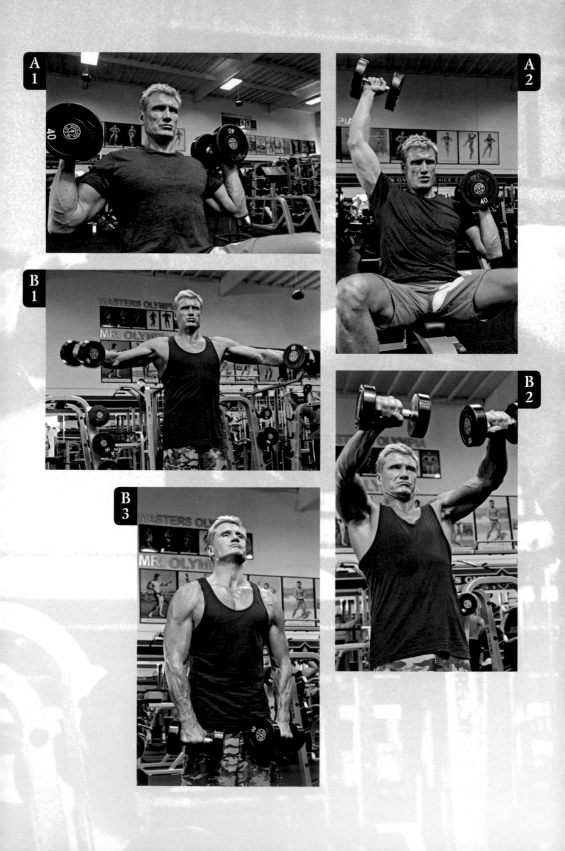

WARM UP
5 minutes on an exercise bicycle, or why not try three minutes "step-up" exercise on a 20-inch bench?

ABDOMINALS
Hanging leg lift
Same exercise as in Program 1. See page 46.

SHOULDERS
"Arnold" dumbbell press
This is my esteemed action colleague "The Governator's" favorite shoulder exercise.

Starting position: Hold the dumbbells at shoulder level with the palms of the hands pointing inward [A1].
Execution: Raise one dumbbell at a time to a straight arm while rotating your hand a one-quarter turn so that the palm faces forward [A2]. This works your entire shoulder girdle effectively.

You can do this exercise both sitting and standing, but standing requires more balance, thereby engaging your core.

Combination shoulder exercise
This has become one of my favorite exercises to get well-developed and symmetrical shoulders.

Starting position: Hold the dumbbells hanging straight down by your thighs.
Execution: Lift the dumbbells straight out to the sides [B1], then bring them forward in an arc until the dumbbells are in front of your face [B2]. Lower the dumbbells to the front of your thighs [B3]. Then reverse the same movement, bringing the dumbbells back up in front of you, out and then down, ending up back in the starting position. This is one repetition. Repeat.

The entire shoulder gets a real challenge with this exercise. It is better to choose a slightly lighter weight and perform the exercise more strictly and deliberately.

ARMS
Standing bicep curl with dumbbells
Starting position: Hold a dumbbell in each hand. Let them hang alongside your body. Tighten your abs.
Execution: Curl one dumbbell until the bicep is fully contracted [A1], then return, controlled, to the starting position. Curl the other dumbbell.

Make sure not to use your hips. Keep your elbows close to your body and focus on your biceps contracting. Warm up with a lighter weight and work your way up.

Concentration curl
This exercise gives your biceps get more peak and definition.

Starting position: Hold a dumbbell in one hand. Support yourself against a bench or dumbbell rack with the other hand.
Execution: Curl the dumbbell slowly until you get a full contraction [B1]. Hold the top position for a beat before slowly returning to the starting position.

The biceps are relatively small muscles and it's important that they do not become over-trained with too many sets and reps for them to grow properly. (I'll do 10–15 sets per workout for my legs, but only 6–10 sets for my biceps.)

Lying triceps press
A classic body builder's "French press," a lying triceps press with dumbbells or a barbell.

Starting position: Hold a barbell with a medium-width grip and lie down on a bench. Raise the barbell until your arms are almost straight [C1].
Execution: Bend your arms and bring the barbell down toward your forehead, until you feel the stretch in the back of your arms [C2]. Return to the top position.

Triceps press on cable machine
This exercise is for you to achieve maximum contraction and definition.

Starting position: Attach a bar to a cable machine. Grip it so you have about six inches between your hands. Lean slightly forward, elbows bent and put one foot behind you for stability.
Execution: Push the bar down until your arms are fully straightened [D1]. Hold for a beat before returning to the starting position. Switch leg position for each set.

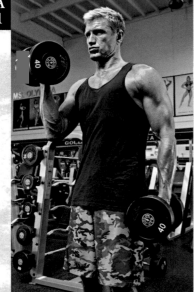

A1

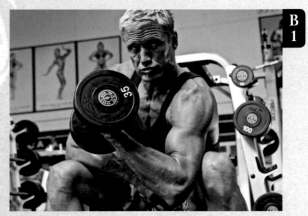

B1

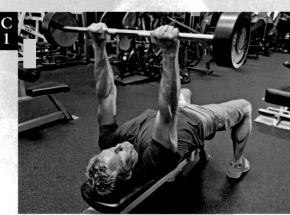

C1

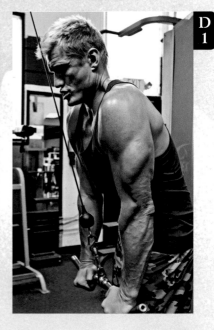

D1

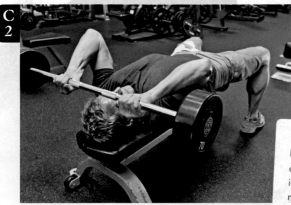

C2

Remember that the triceps are larger than your biceps, so in order to get beefy arms it's important not to neglect this muscle!

LOWER BACK/ABDOMINALS
Back lifts/sit-ups on the ball
Back lift
See page 48.

Sit-ups on the Swiss ball
Starting position: Lie with your lower back on a Swiss ball and your feet firmly on the floor [A1].
Execution: Raise your upper body as far as you can [A2] and return, controlled, to the starting position.

You can vary this exercise by raising up your upper body diagonally, engaging the sides of your torso and abdominal muscles.

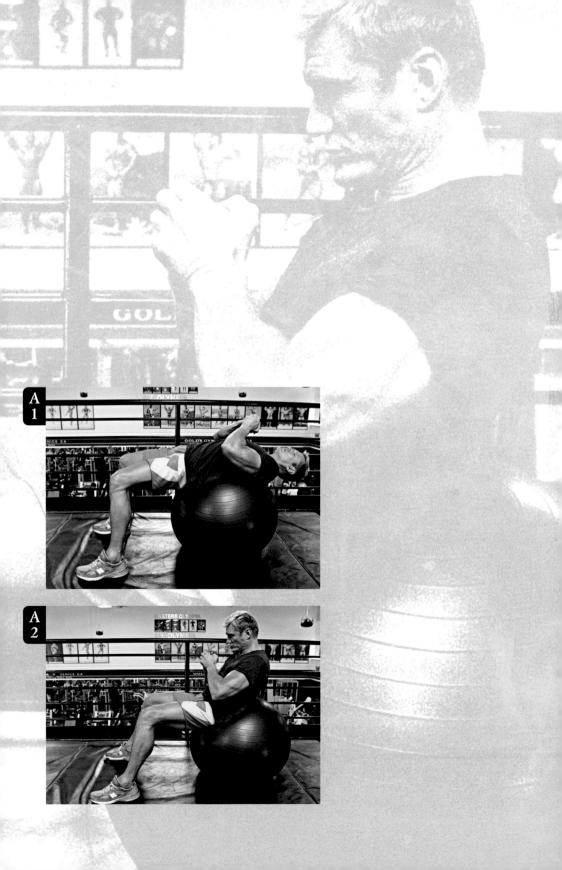

STRETCH
DL stretch (see page 110).

CARDIO
Shadowboxing, punching bag, or jumping jacks. (Also see No Excuses on page 126.)

Total time for DL Program 3: 45 minutes

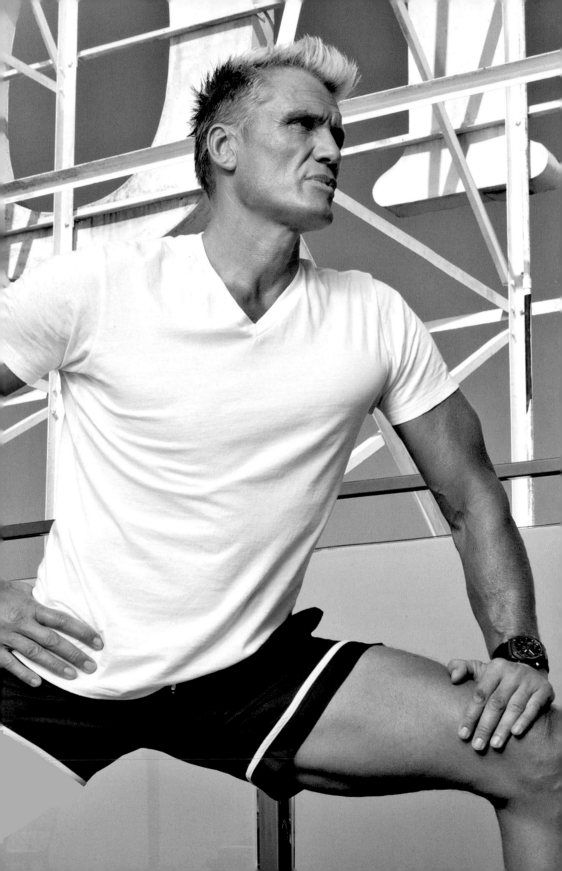

Here's a workout that trains the entire body and also increases your aerobic capacity. Circuit training regimens are often used by MMA fighters and by special military units.

A perfect workout if you can only train once or twice a week and want to work the whole body.

Keep your intensity high during this workout and don't go too heavy.

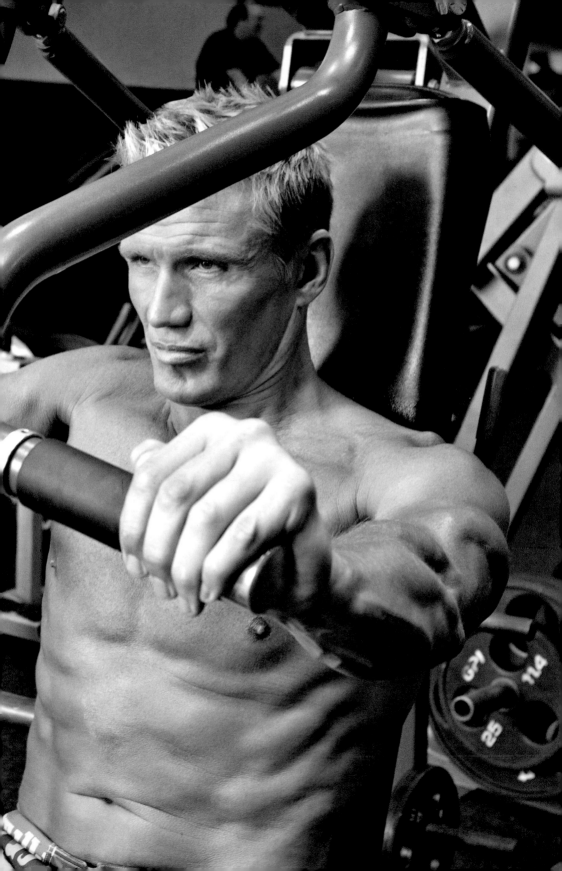

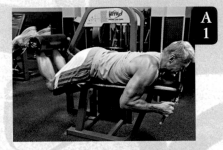

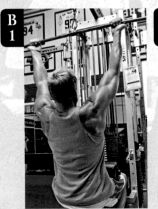

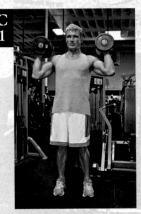

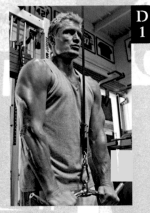

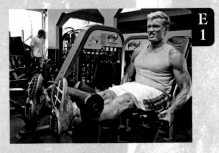

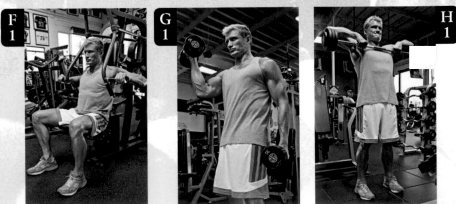

WARM UP
3 minutes on the exercise bike with low resistance.

CIRCUIT 1
Leg curls (15 reps) [A1]: See page 62
Lat pulls (15 reps) [B1]: See page 68
"Arnold" dumbbell press (15 reps) [C1]: See page 75
Triceps press on the cable machine (15 reps) [D1]: See page 76

NOTE: No rest between these four sets then back on the bike.

Keep moving throughout all exercises in Circuit 1. When you get back to the bike, you get to rest your muscles for 3 minutes, but you still get a cardio workout.

Exercise bike: 3 minutes at low resistance.

Repeat Circuit 1: Perform the four weight exercises and go back to the exercise bike.

Exercise bike: 3 minutes at medium resistance.

CIRCUIT 2
Leg extensions (15 reps) [E1]: See page 48
Chest press machine (15 reps) [F1]: See page 90
Standing bicep curls with dumbbells (12 reps, left/right) [G1]: See page 76
Upright row (15 reps) [H1]: See page 89

NOTE: No rest between sets then back on the bike

Exercise bike: 3 minutes at medium resistance.

Repeat Circuit 2: Perform the four weight exercises and go back to the exercise bike.

Exercise bike: 3 minutes at high resistance.

CIRCUIT 3
Leg press machine (15 reps) [A1]: See page 51
Seated row machine (15 reps) [B1]: See page 68
Lateral dumbbell raises (15 reps) [C1]: See page 89
Pec-deck (15 reps) [D1]: See page 90

Exercise bike: 3 minutes at high resistance.

Repeat Circuit 3: Perform the four weight exercises then back on the bike.

Rest for 2 minutes.

You have done Circuit 1 twice, Circuit 2 twice, and Circuit 3 twice, for a total of six circuits, with a 3-minute break on the exercise bike between each circuit.

ABDOMINALS
Perform this sequence three times without rest: 20 seconds plank, 10 push-ups, 20 seconds side plank on the right side, 10 push-ups, 20 seconds side plank on the left side, 10 push-ups [E1-3].

STRETCH
DL Stretch (see page 110). 3 minutes.

CARDIO
2 minutes shadowboxing.

Total time for DL Program 4: 60 minutes

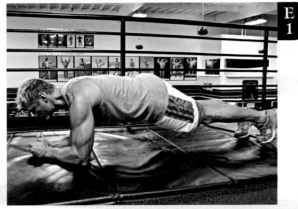

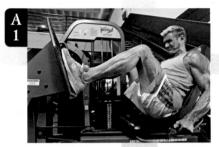

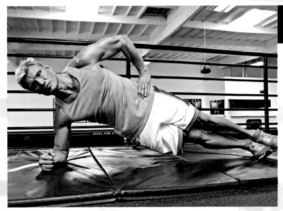

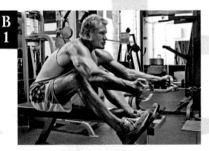

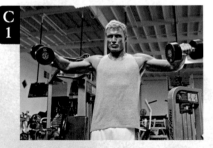

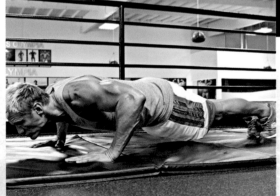

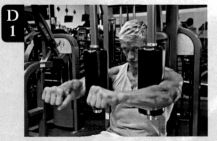

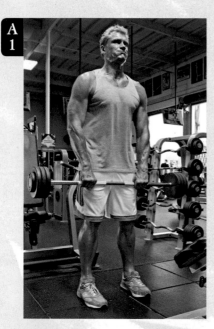

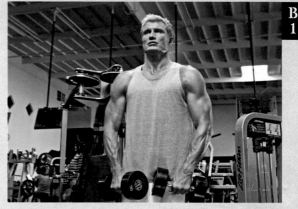

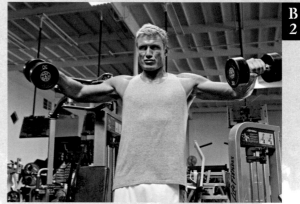

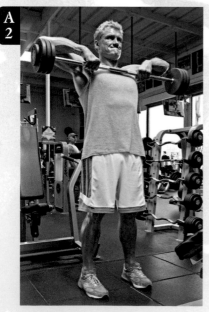

NEW EXERCISES IN DL PROGRAM 4

SHOULDERS
Upright row
Starting position: Grip a barbell with a shoulder-width grip. Tighten your abs and stand up straight [A1].
Execution: Raise the bar to your chin with your elbows pointing up and outward [A2]. Return, controlled, to the starting position.

Lateral dumbbell raises
Starting position: Hold a dumbbell in each hand. Tighten your abs, keeping your core stable [B1].
Execution: Raise the dumbbells with your arms slightly bent until your arms are parallel to the floor [B2]. Return, controlled, to the starting position.

NEW EXERCISES IN DL PROGRAM 4

CHEST
Pec-deck and chest press machine
Pec-deck
Starting position: Sit on a pec-deck machine with the seat high enough that your upper arms are parallel to the floor. Make sure your forearms are against the cushions [A1].
Execution: Pull your forearms forward and inward, bringing the cushions together in front of you. Hold this position for a beat before returning, controlled, to the starting position [A2].

Chest press machine
Starting position: Sit on a chest press machine and adjust the seat so that your chest is in line with the grips [B1].
Execution: Gripping the handles with your shoulders lowered, steadily press the handles forward until your arms are almost fully extended. Return, controlled, to the starting position.

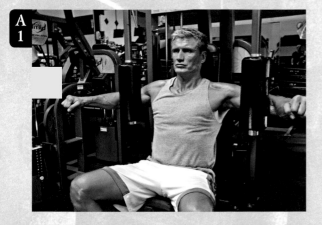

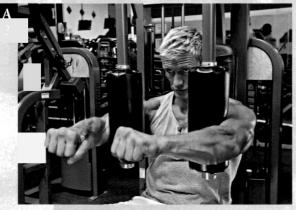

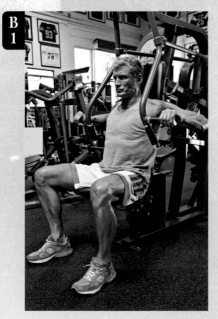

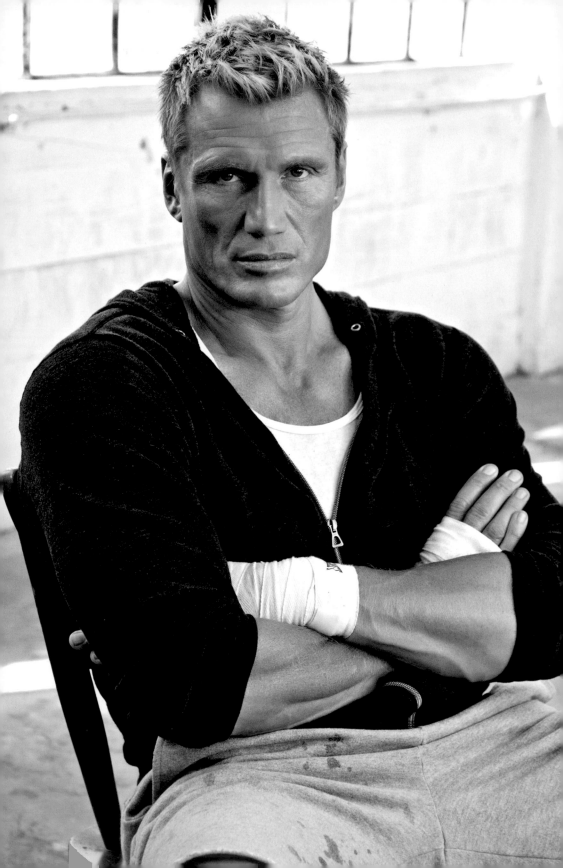

ENDURANCE TRAINING

Aerobic exercises like karate, running, cycling, and swimming are an important part of any training regimen. How much cardio I do depends on how my body is feeling and what type of project I'm working on. If I have a karate training camp coming up where I have to spar every day, my workouts will consist of more cardio and less strength. If I'm making a film where I have to look extra muscular, like *The Expendables*, I'll do more strength training and endurance becomes secondary.

When I started training, endurance-type training dominated. From about age fifteen, my physical exercise consisted of ice hockey, martial arts, and a bit of weight training.

When you practice karate, speed and endurance are the most important tools for success. I added strength training as a supplement when I started competing. I used weights mainly to build strength and power, especially during the off-season phase.

When I first came to Hollywood it was very important *how* my body looked. So I took on more serious bodybuilding. I started learning about different routines put together weight workouts that later became an important part of my Fully Integrated Training System, "FIT."

FIT is based on weight training, but it also includes exercises for your endurance and flexibility. Better endurance not only makes you feel good, it also provides the stamina needed to perform longer and tougher strength training workouts. Better endurance has also been shown to help combat stress. Stretching will make your body less susceptible to injury. In Chapter 6, Tactics, you will learn how to combine all the pieces of this puzzle for a successful training schedule.

Look for your own balance between strength and endurance. Personally, I've found that it works well to follow a training program with approximately sixty percent focus on muscle strength and forty percent on aerobic fitness.

TRAINING INTENSITY

In competitive sports, the physical intensity varies greatly throughout the match or a game. Whether it's football, hockey, or racket sports, first you're on the offensive, then you're defending, taking time out, or giving it that supreme effort to reach the finish line. This certainly applies to martial arts. Varying the intensity is something you should keep in mind when planning your training.

When you combine the exercise bike or running on a treadmill with weight training in the gym, you get a double training effect. Your muscles keep working in a new capacity while recovering from the previous type of training. In martial arts, this effect is true when you spar. A fight may start with tactical long-range sniping and end as a slugfest.

Focusing on varying the intensity led me to include the circuit workout in DL Program 4, combining strength training and aerobic exercise.

In that workout, the goal is to keep your heart rate at fifty to sixty percent of your maximum level, reaching up to seventy to eighty percent during the aerobic portions of the program.

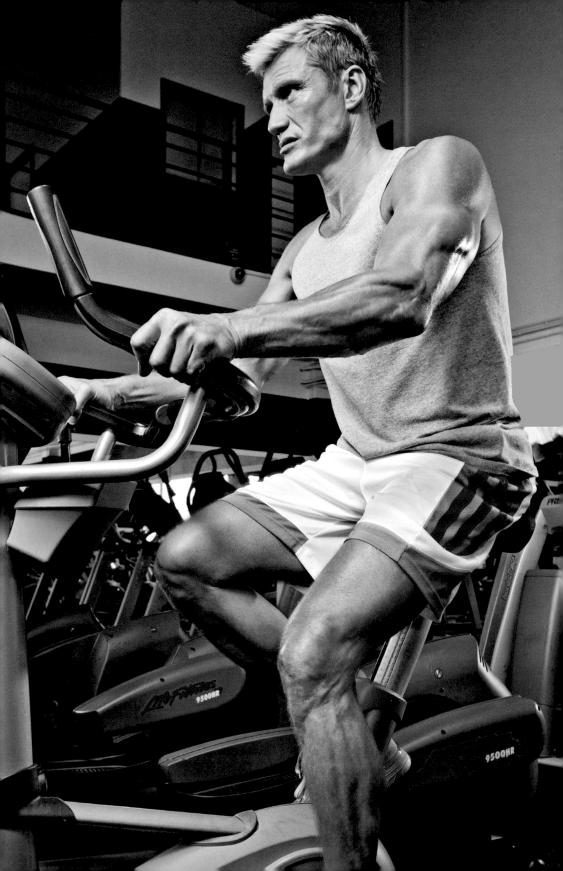

MARTIAL ARTS TRAINING—MORE THAN JUST CARDIO

To me, the martial arts are the most versatile and stimulating form of exercise. Boxing and karate both express a particular human impulse: the struggle for survival. This impulse is deeply embedded in our genetic code and gives us an extra adrenaline kick when we face down an opponent or even a heavy punching bag.

In addition, continuing to work on your coordination skills ensures that your body will stay functional. Punching and kicking combinations keep your neural circuits alert. Plus you can defend yourself should the need arise (see DL Self Defense System at the end of each chapter). Martial arts and boxing increase your aerobic fitness and burn fat more effectively than many other forms of endurance training.

Like most combat sports, it's more satisfying when you train with a partner.

Martial arts and boxing build self-confidence and a humility that is "hard to beat." I hope you get the chance to try out some of the martial arts workouts in this book. Try this type of training as a warm-up in the cardio parts of your training sessions.

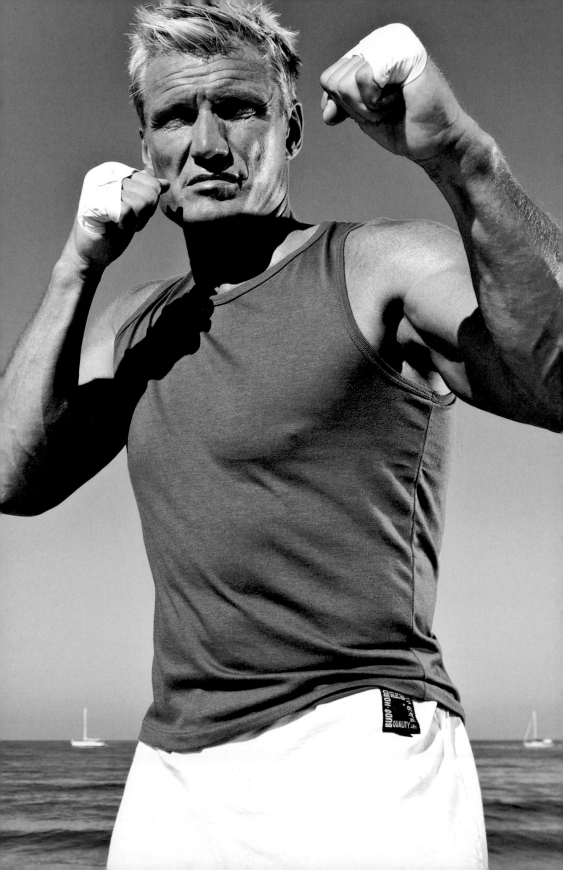

MARTIAL ARTS EXERCISES

Here are some basic exercises that you can use as a warm up or as a complete cardio workout. You can also combine a treadmill running workout with a couple of rounds of shadowboxing, or go five rounds on the heavy bag and then do my No Excuses routine, with push-ups, sit-ups, squats, and so on.

Normal rest between 3-minute rounds is one minute. For 2-minute rounds, rest 30 seconds.

Shadowboxing

Shadowboxing is a classic exercise that you can do anywhere, preferably in front of a mirror.

Try out these basic boxing techniques:
• Left jab [A1]
• Right cross [A2]
• Left hook [A3]
• Uppercut to the body or to the head [A4]
(Switch hands if you are a "southpaw," i.e. leading with your right)

Move your upper body from side to side while staying light on your feet. "Float like a butterfly, sting like a bee!" said heavyweight champion Muhammad Ali.

Try skipping rope to warm up. A three-minute round skipping rope is like jogging for ten minutes. It's better to start with a two-minute round and work your way up to three minutes, both with skipping rope and shadowboxing. Shadowboxing is particularly great as a cool down after a hard strength workout. It helps your body and prevents muscle soreness.

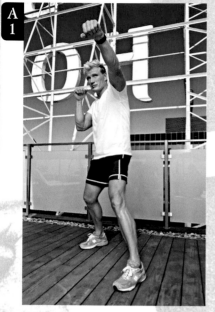

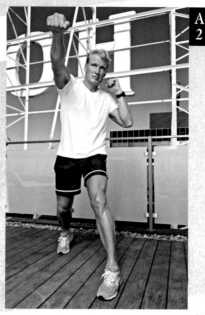

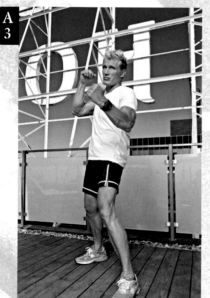

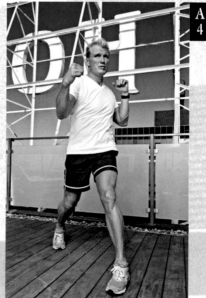

100

MARTIAL ARTS EXERCISES
Heavy bag

Many gyms today have heavy bags. If your gym has an instructor-led session, all you need to do is sign up, but sometimes it can be nice to test it out for yourself. Use regular boxing gloves or special bag gloves that are a bit lighter, but still protect your hands. Assume a boxing stance in front of the bag. Move back and forth, then circle left and right while throwing the punches described above. You can also try a couple of karate techniques. The easiest is the knee kick, where you hit the target with the upper side of your knee. The front kick is using the ball of your foot to strike the target. Try using the elbow when close to the bag to vary your workouts.

Start slowly practicing in front of the mirror and work your way to hitting a heavy bag. Keep your punches and kicks quick and sharp. To use Mohammed Ali's words: it's that "bee sting" we're after!

Striking Pads

You can combine all three of these exercises, for example:

DL Knockout

One round (2 minutes) skipping rope
Three rounds with the striking pads
Three rounds on the heavy bag
Push-ups (maximum number in one minute)
Sit-ups (maximum number in one minute)
Squats (maximum number in one minute)
One round skipping rope
Stretching

Total time: 30 minutes of effective training

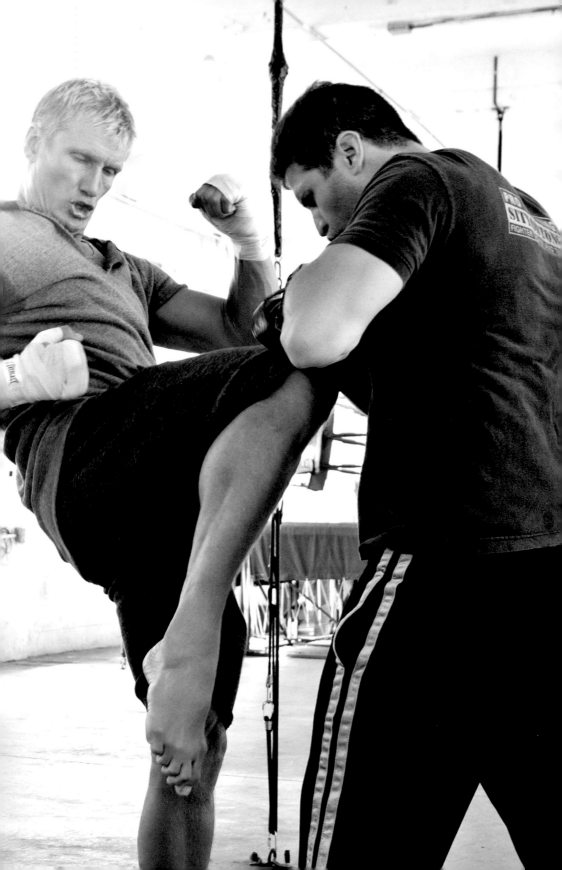

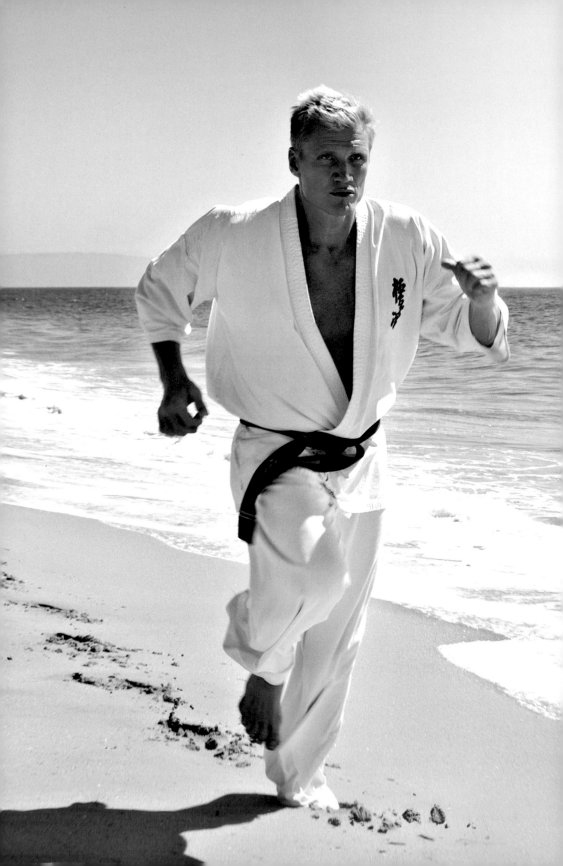

RUNNING—THE ORIGINAL EXERCISE

Thousands of years ago, the human hunter-gatherer's body had to walk long distances. He or she had to run if threatened or to bring down game. Walking and running are the original and most basic exercises for the human body. I love walking and make running part of my endurance training, but in short doses. When you weigh 230 pounds, your body isn't really built for long-distance running. I must have been the guy with the stone axe who waited to ambush the game!

If I run more than three miles I feel it the next day, especially if running on a hard surface. I prefer wind sprints on the beach or the treadmill set on a three percent incline. Otherwise, it's a long walk in the morning—a great way to regroup, burn fat, and gather your thoughts. If you're a running buff, then you have a great way to burn fat and build your aerobic fitness.

Interval training on the treadmill is my favorite—less boring and more effective. I usually do thirty seconds of jogging and then thirty seconds of harder pace and so on for fifteen to twenty minutes. I prefer to be outdoors, running the same intervals up a hill. If you're at a hotel, doing the stairs is also great. Climbing stairs at a walk or run is a simple and effective way to build leg strength as well as aerobic fitness.

Running is probably the best and easiest way to achieve good basic fitness. Just remember to get a good pair of running shoes and special insoles if needed, especially if you weigh a little extra like I do!

SWIMMING

I love swimming. When I travel, I usually check if they have a pool at the hotel where I'm staying. I pack goggles and swim trunks, looking forward to some good workouts during my stay.

Swimming is, along with cross-country skiing, arguably the least damaging and most effective all-round exercise you can do. The whole body is put to work in a gentle combination of calisthenics and aerobics.

Ideally you should have access to pool that's not too short. It gets a little monotonous doing fifty to a hundred laps in a twenty-five foot pool, turning around every seven seconds.

The fitness guru Jack LaLanne (who lived to ninety-six years of age) advocated swimming as "The Greatest Exercise." As a sixty-year-old
(in 1974), with his hands and feet tied, LaLanne swam from Alcatraz Island to San Francisco's Fisherman's Wharf, towing a 1,000-pound boat behind him. The water wasn't exactly lukewarm and the man wasn't wearing a wetsuit.

No one today could replicate this feat, possibly with the exception of Ivan Drago.

DL SWIM
There are two swimming workouts I like to do, especially when I am traveling. The first is a little easier, the other slightly more demanding.

Dolphin 1
Swim one length (25 meters) breaststroke, turn, and crawl back. Repeat for 500 meters. Then do as many push-ups as possible in one minute, then a minute of sit-ups, and finally a minute of squats. Stretch.

Dolphin 2
Warm up by swimming 200 meters at an easy pace (100 meters breaststroke, 100 meters crawl). Then do the following sprint series:
• 4 x 100 meter crawl (resting 1 minute between each sprint)
• 4 x 50 meter crawl (resting 30 seconds between each sprint)
• 4 x 25 meter crawl (resting 15 seconds between each sprint)
Cool down by swimming 50 meters backstroke and 50 meters breaststroke at an easy pace.
Total distance: 1000 meters.

Finish by stretching.

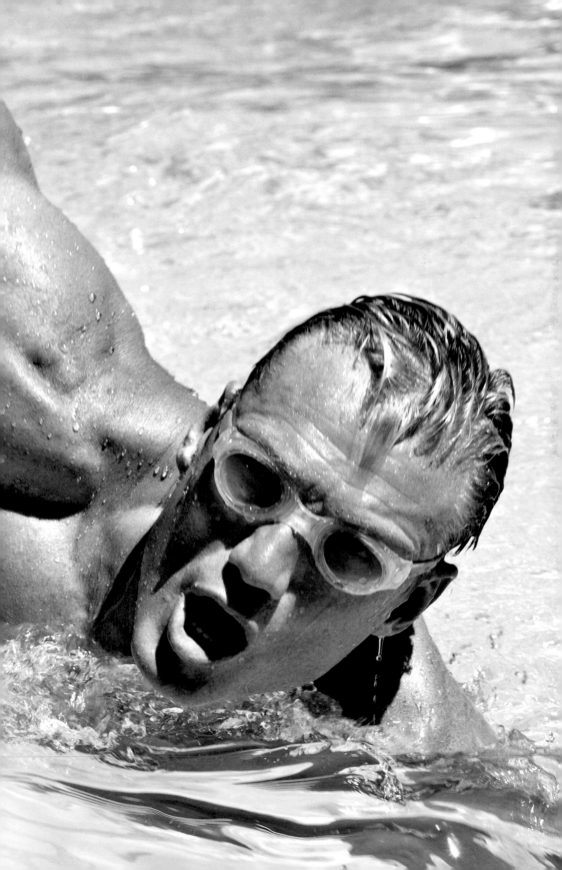

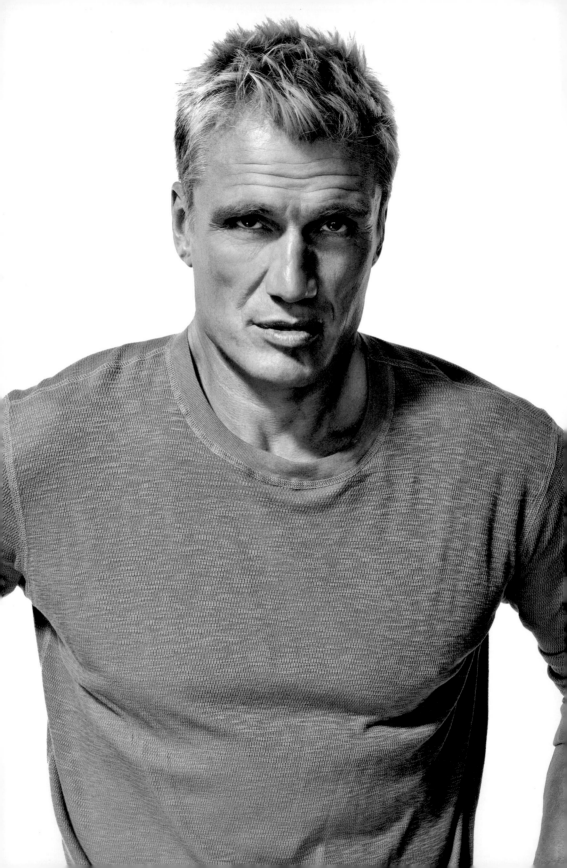

STRETCHING, RELAXATION, AND MEDITATION

Flexibility is paramount in order to maintain a functional physique. If you do strength and endurance training regularly, but neglect flexibility you could be more prone to athletic injuries. The lower back, hip flexors, shoulders, and hamstrings are potential problem areas for many people involved in physical training.

The older I get, the more I realize how important mobility is. I've included stretching and flexibility training in all of my workout programs. Even if I have the day off from training, I make sure to stretch.

Stretching keeps your body young.

Normally I stretch first thing in the morning, before breakfast, usually after ten minutes of meditation. I also stretch after my strength and endurance workouts (see DL Stretch on page 110). My karate training and my home workouts also contain some flexibility exercises.

Stretching creates excellent muscle awareness and it's also relaxing. It opens up the energy pathways in the body, relieving tension and problem areas in your body.

It's a good way to reduce muscle soreness and speed up the recovery process after hard exercise.

IF EXERCISE IS SILVER, THEN REST IS GOLD

It isn't the workout that builds your body; rather, it's during the resting phase that your muscle fibers thicken to deal with the next training session. Proper sleep and relaxation for your body to recuperate are very important when you plan a long-term training schedule.

An ambitious career, the Internet and a packed agenda can easily chip away at your time for rest and recovery. Train too hard without rest and you'll become over-trained, lose muscle mass, and expose yourself to a greater risk of injury.

Don't try to keep the same workout pace week in, week out. Take a week off from training.

If you take five to seven days off from training, you'll feel eager to get going again. A rest period also provides a little extra time to evaluate your training results. It gives you the time to become curious about new exercises and to plan new training regimens.

Remember to take it easy when you first get back in the gym.

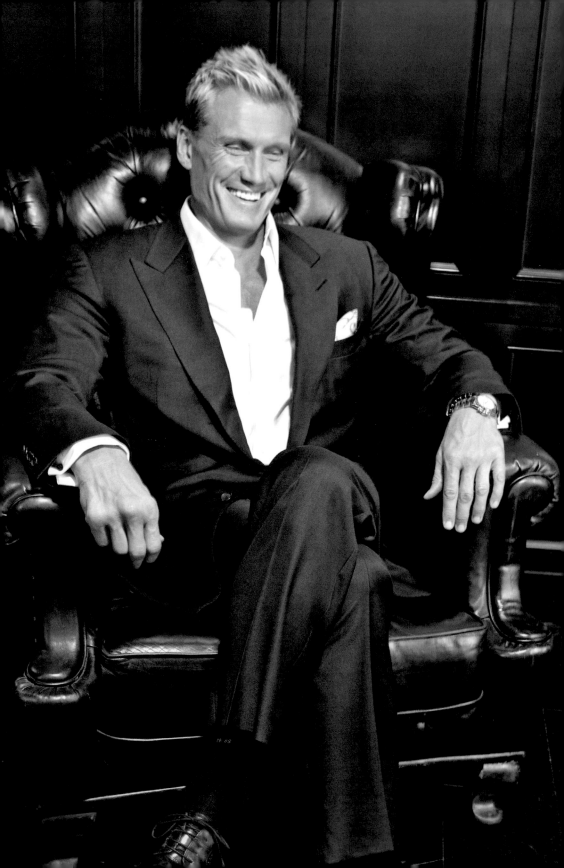

More on rest and meditation: Sometimes I try to force myself to just do nothing, just stay at home all day. Especially, if I've finished a busy period of work and I need time to unwind. I try not to do much at all, just to be alone with myself and my thoughts sounds like enough to do for a whole day. It's more rewarding than you may think.

Let your *body* and *mind* catch up to each other.

Read more about meditation in the next chapter, Special Ops.

I try to get a deep-tissue massage at least once a week. It gives me a moment of mental relaxation and helps my muscle recovery. I believe that regular massage is beneficial for the internal balance of the whole body. It helps to remove waste products from the muscles and brings the body's energy pathways into balance. We all have a strong need to feel human touch. In many Eastern cultures, receiving massages is a natural part of a person's overall body consciousness. The West should follow their lead more. The former actor and comedian Bob Hope got a massage every day from his thirties until his death. Hope was as sharp as a tack at age eighty-two when I worked with him and he lived to be one hundred years old.

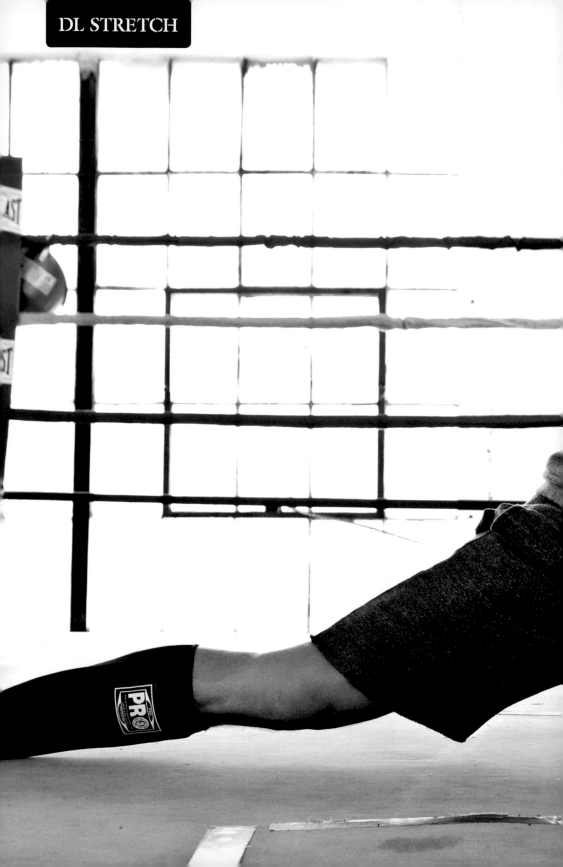

DL STRETCH

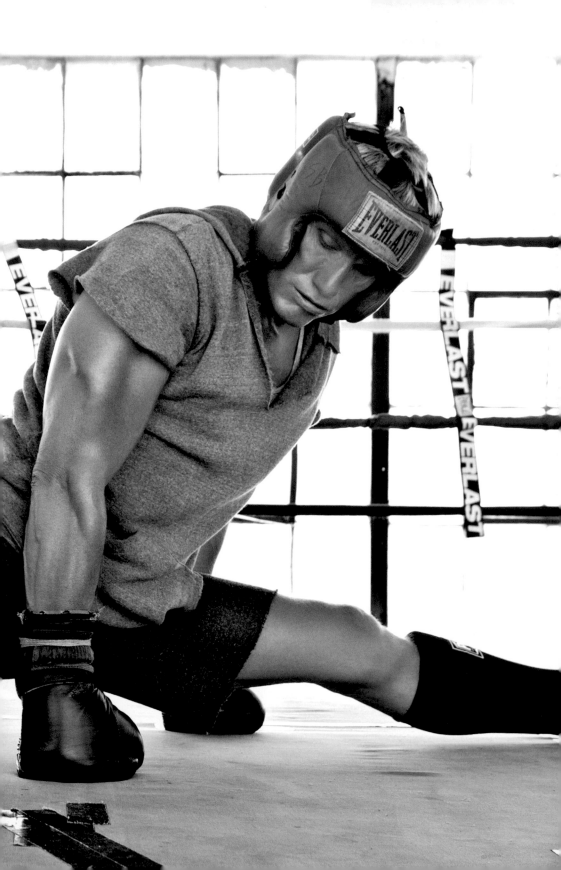

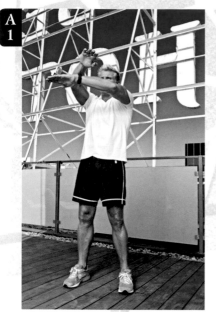

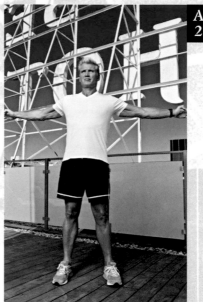

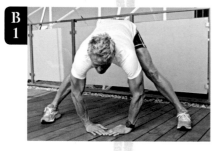

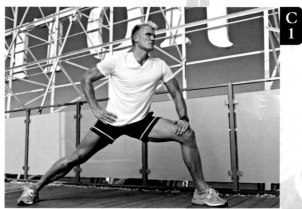

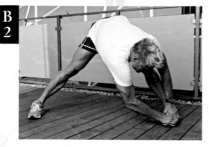

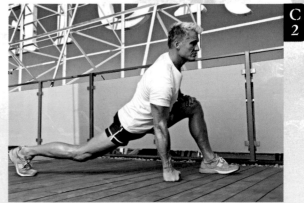

Arm rotations
Stand relaxed with your feet hip-width apart. Keep your arms slightly bent and rotate them five times forward [A1] then five times in the opposite direction [A2].

Karate stretch for hips and legs: front/left/right
Stand with your feet two shoulder-widths apart. Bend your upper body forward and downward toward the floor. Drop your elbows and stretch your thighs and back for 10 seconds [B1]. Bring your upper body toward your left leg and hold for 10 seconds [B2]. Repeat with the right leg.

Karate stretch for inner thighs and hip flexors
Stand with your feet two shoulder-widths apart. Bend your left knee and lean your body to the left, stretching the inside of the right leg [C1]. Hold for 10 seconds. Then turn your feet and hips all the way to the left and drop your knee further, stretching the right hip flexor. Put one hand on the floor for balance and a better stretch [C2]. Repeat on the right side.

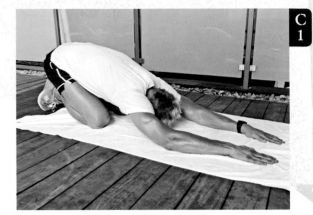

C1

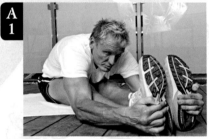

A1

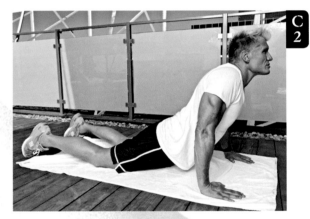

C2

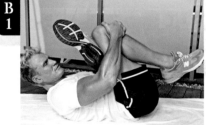

B1

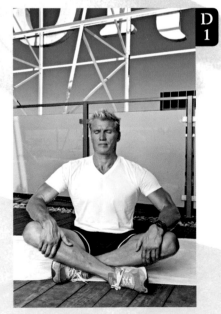

D1

Seated stretch for hamstrings

Sit down with your legs straight in front of you, keeping your knees and ankles together. Lower your upper body toward your knees. Hold for 10 seconds [A1].

Stretch for buttocks

Lie on your back. Using your hands, take hold of your leg and bend the knee, facing the knee away from your body. Place your other knee behind the foot for a greater stretch. Pull the leg toward you for 10 seconds [B1]. Repeat with the other leg.

Stretch for the abdominals and lower back

Kneel. Extend your arms in front of you, as you slide your hips back and lower your body toward your thighs [C1]. Hold for 10 seconds. Then extend your upper body forward and upward, dropping your hips, supporting your body with your hands on the floor. Keep your gaze directed upward [C2]. Hold for 10 seconds.

Seated meditation

Sit relaxed, cross-legged. Close your eyes and breathe in through your nose, deep into the stomach and then exhale through a half-open mouth. Focus on your breathing. Feel each breath, the coolness in your nose, how your chest and stomach expand. Try not to think about anything other than your breathing [D1].

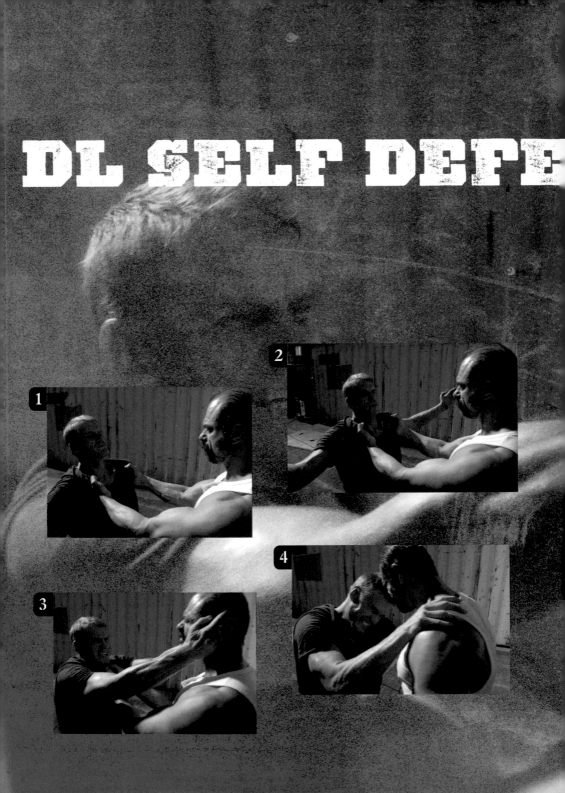

AGAINST A FRONTAL GRAB

Use your cupped hands to rupture the assailant's eardrums [2 and 3].
Follow up with a head butt [4].

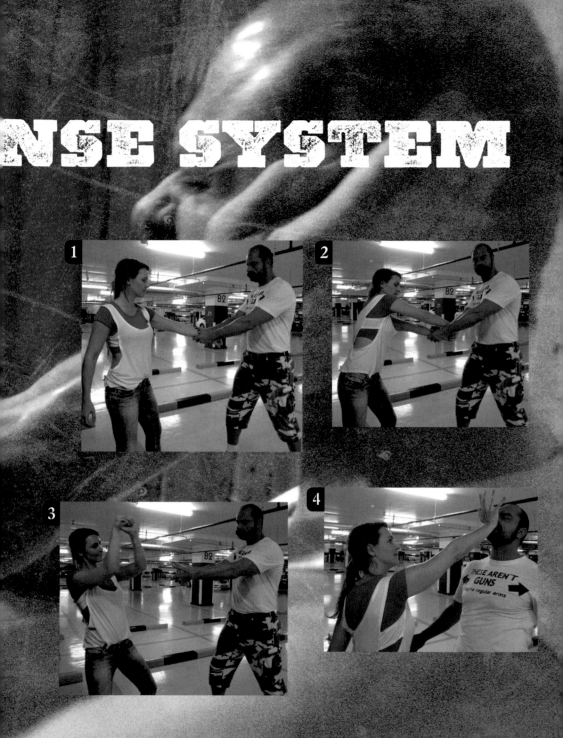

NSE SYSTEM

AGAINST A DOUBLE-HANDED GRAB

Grab your own wrist with the other hand and pull up and back against the assailant's thumbs—the weakest part of any grip [2].
Follow up with a palm heel strike to the nose [4].

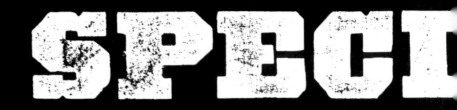

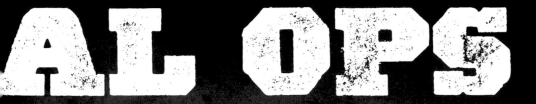

TRAINING UNDER EXTREME CONDITIONS

Sometimes you end up in situations that are not favorable for training. Life doesn't always play by your rules. Using my training regimen, you can still stay in good shape. You don't have to go to the gym to get an effective workout!

The film industry is an international industry. My life as an actor requires an immense amount of travel each year. Before each film project begins, business contacts must be established, financing must be found, and shooting locations have to be tracked down. Once filming is underway it often takes place in a variety of places, sometimes on different continents.

The release of the film once again requires whirlwind publicity tours between countries for interviews, television shows, and promotional assignments.

Sometimes I wake up in a hotel bed wondering which movie I'm promoting and where!

When I first started out in the industry, the rapid pace came as a shock. I realized how difficult it was to stick to anything that resembled a training schedule. I was used to having sufficient time for my workout routines, but as the film projects became more frequent and demanding, the time available for training diminished.

I began to notice how worn out I became from the constant travel, irregular hours, and inadequate training.

Even if you don't work in the film industry, you've probably experienced this problem. With too much work, it's difficult to keep to any schedule. This is particularly true of exercise. Working irregular hours at home, your normal gym routines can easily be neglected.

Training "on the move" is a challenge to both your creativity and planning.

In my early twenties I received a scholarship from the Royal Institute of Technology in Sweden to finish my chemical engineering education at Sydney University in Australia. With my parents, my siblings, and my home country left behind, I had truly begun my journey into the wide world. I didn't know it then, but my farewell to Sweden would be considerably longer than one academic year. Soon, my life was to change more than I'd ever imagined.

I had received a scholarship to Sydney University for two academic terms to finish my Masters degree. Thoughts of what would I would do afterward were already swirling around in my head. I had a far-reaching plan of continuing my studies in the United States, first to get a PhD in engineering, then to proceed to a top business school, like Harvard or MIT. Like my older brother, I wanted to work in the petroleum industry. However, sitting on that airplane on my way to Australia, work and career were still far beyond the horizon and I felt no great need to reflect on them.

I landed at Sydney Airport on a sunny Sunday morning, took the bus into the city, and dragged my incredibly heavy suitcase from the bus station through half-empty streets to the university's red administrative buildings. It was hard to believe that I was on the other side of the world.

When the plane had taken off from the Stockholm airport it was winter, but "down-under" in Sydney it was high summer.

I tried my hardest to fit in to campus life, but it was not as easy as when I was studying in the US. The American kids at Washington State seemed to me more open and curious about foreigners than the more reserved people of Australia.

For the first time since I moved from home to northern Sweden, I felt alone.

I focused on my work.

Academics and sports became my life.

The university offered good workout opportunities and I quickly started my "own" karate club for interested students. We trained hard every night. While at it, I won the Australian Open Championship and the Sydney Team Championships. Finally, I also began to find some friends through karate. Unfortunately, as usual I didn't find any girlfriends.

I sparred with my friend Mark, an ex-boxer who was big and damn tough. A good thing for me, because the Australian Open Championship roster included a local heavyweight champion who boasted of how he would sweep the floor with that "f . . . ing Swede." The final was tough because of his physical size, but my experience and stamina soon took its toll. He collapsed after a few minutes and I was declared the winner by *ippon*, or a knock-out. When I met the guy five years later during my PR tour for a film, it seemed like he was still limping from my repeated "low kicks" against his left thigh.

I did weight training after my karate sessions, mainly for strength and explosiveness. It was noticeable not only in my competitions but also on my body. I had begun to resemble a young Steve Reeves.

My academic work went well. After completing my studies in Australia, I applied for a scholarship to attend one of the world's leading technical universities, Massachusetts Institute of Technology, better known as MIT. All according to plan.

MIT was the school that my dad had always talked about. His dream.

I couldn't fail a class or drop a grade if I was to be accepted to MIT. I studied like a madman. I had to graduate at the top of my class at Sydney University to get the Fulbright Scholarship I needed to pay for my studies at MIT.

A top student from China and I would compete for first place.

Training and studying finally took its toll and I caught a serious flu from physical exhaustion and psychological stress. Luckily, my training had made me strong and I soon recovered.

Student life is seldom lucrative, so when the opportunity came along to make some extra cash, I took it. It wasn't unknown to the people around me that I trained and competed in karate. One day my workout buddy Mark and I received an employment proposition: There were rock concerts being held in an arena in Sydney and the organizers needed security for the artists. We would act as bodyguards during the concerts and afterward when the performers did their tour of the Sydney nightlife.

It was impossible to say no to ten Australian dollars an hour.

The third musketeer in our security team was "Doc" John, who was a fixture at all karate competitions in Sydney. "Doc" was not a real doctor, but an ex-medical student who, a few years earlier had decided to make some extra cash by making amphetamines in his garage and selling them to locals. He fell headlong down that road, spent some time on the inside. Now he was back on the straight and narrow. I had accidentally broken his nose during one of our sparring sessions and thought it was only right that he also benefit from this new gravy train.

On a side note, "Doc" John has long since earned back his license to practice medicine. He has become a renowned researcher on the treatment of drug addicts and lectures on this subject throughout the world. Good on you, John!

I stood there half asleep and listened to the various superstars of the eighties. There were artists such as Doctor Hook, David Bowie, Joan Armatrading, and the New York disco queen Grace Jones.

When Grace arrived in Sydney on her world tour, my karate buddies and I were appointed her personal bodyguards. First outside her dressing room and later keeping her overly excited fans at a distance at the after party. That there would be serious partying later with a "Studio 54" icon like Grace Jones was guaranteed.

Grace immediately appointed the tall, blonde Swede as her special close protector. I did my best to give her as much security as possible in the various nightclubs she visited with her entourage. It didn't take many hours before we had taken a liking to each other.

Grace was a very special lady and I was charmed by her half-crazy manner and New York style. Why she fell for me, I can only guess. It probably had something do with my Steve Reeves physique.

The evening ended with an invitation to her hotel suite for a drink. I missed my first class in the morning.

Although Grace left Australia a short while later, we had started a relationship that would mean the beginning of a complete change in my life. ○

> **THE EVENING ENDED WITH AN INVITATION TO HER HOTEL ROOM . . . AND THE REST IS HISTORY.**

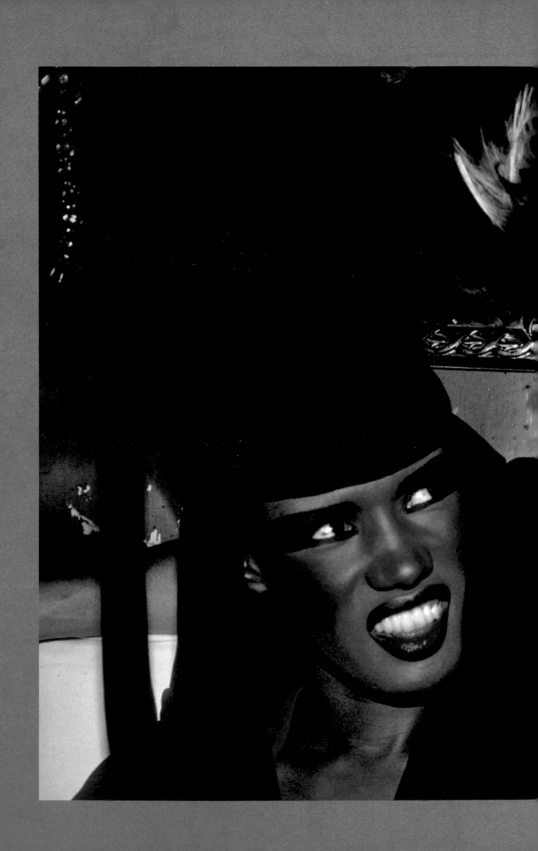

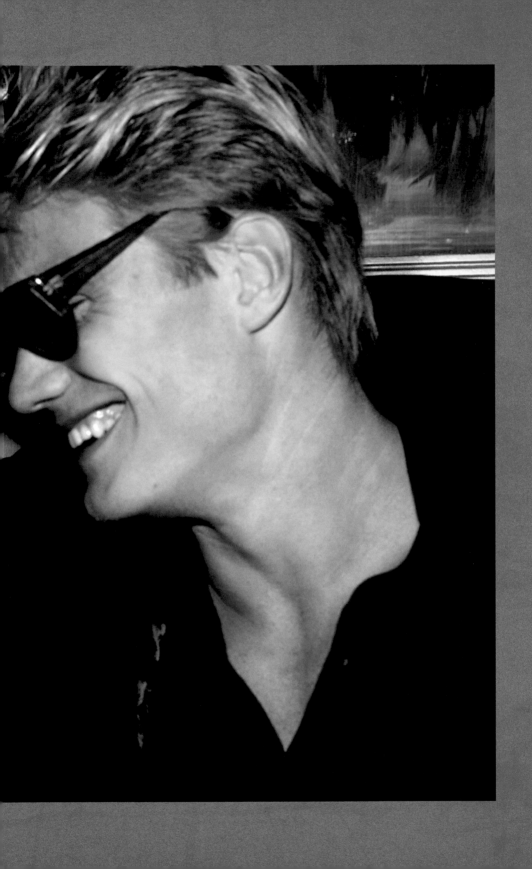

"Excuse me, is there a gym around here . . .?" When I go filming around the world there are usually good gyms nearby, but it still doesn't solve the exercise issue. Finding time to work out every day can difficult. The logistics of a film production are often very hectic and the shooting schedule constantly changes because of weather, technical problems, etc.

Plans and routines have to be adjusted. It can be difficult to find time for long workouts in the gym.

I distinctly remember one production in Toronto where we started filming very early every morning. I decided to work out despite the extreme working hours. So I got up at 3:15 *in the morning* to get a session in between 3:30 and 4:30 a.m. I came home from training, had breakfast, and was picked up at 5:30. Yeah, I like morning workouts, but that was a little too exhausting!

It is on these types of experiences that my special workout routines in this chapter are based.

TIME TO TRAIN—WHEN YOU DON'T HAVE THE TIME

When I first entered the film industry, my physique suffered from not getting a chance to train properly. My workouts were gym-based and mostly based around using weights. I decided to develop additional workout routines that didn't require a fully equipped gym or lots of time. To create complete workouts that can be done in as little as fifteen minutes and still have an impact.

I'm talking about the No Excuses programs.

I experimented for several years, trying different variations and combinations of exercises. The goal was to create programs for total body workouts that could be done anywhere, no matter what equipment was available.

I regularly supplement my own training with these routines. If there's a pool around, I'll combine a swim with one of these No Excuses workouts.

If you're busy, the mornings are a good time to do these programs. You get a full-body workout, grab a shower, and then a nice breakfast. A great start to a busy day!

This program eliminates all excuses for not exercising, ergo No Excuses!

> **SPECIAL OPS TRAINING**
>
> **Three smart tips when you don't have the time**
>
> 1. Be realistic with your fitness goals.
> 2. If you are not going to the gym, do a shorter program at home. Anything is better than nothing!
> 3. When you're being pressed for time and energy, try to cover at least TWO of the THREE essential components of staying in shape:
>   Exercise, Nutrition, and Sleep.

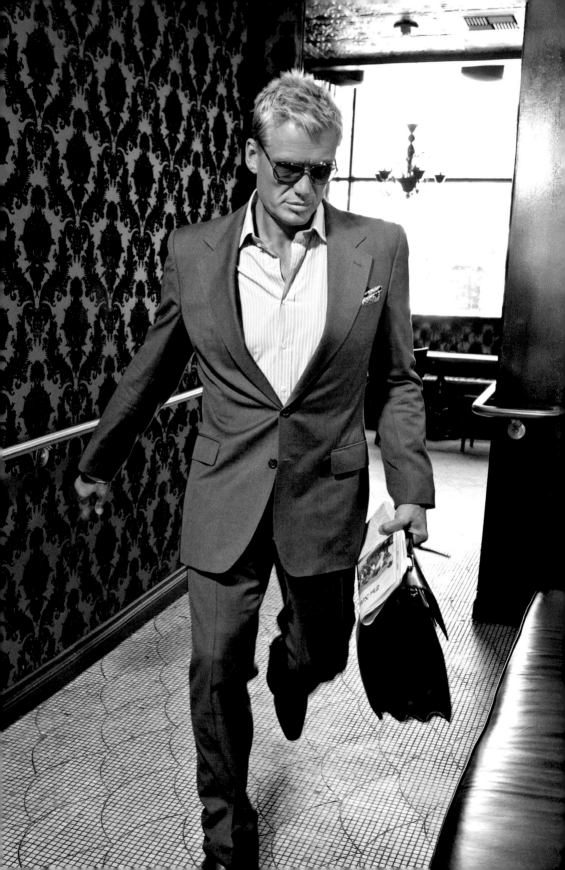

15 MINUTES

This short workout program was inspired by US Navy SEAL fitness routines and my karate workouts. It can be done without weights or equipment. The only thing you need is a sturdy door to do half-chins.

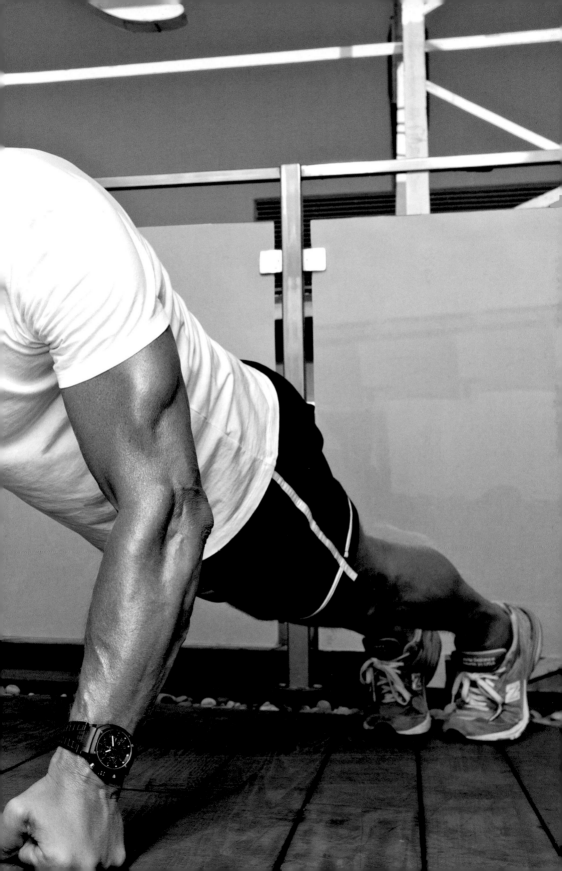

WARM UP

Warm up for 2 minutes with exercises like shadow boxing, high knees, jumping jacks, or skipping rope. The important thing is that you get your heart rate up and get ready for the exercises.

TRAINING BLOCK
Military Eight-Step Exercise (10 times)

This is a US Navy SEAL exercise that gets the whole body up and running.

Starting position: Stand straight with your eyes looking straight ahead, feet together, and hands at your sides [A1]
Execution: Bend your knees and place both hands flat on the floor with your eyes forward [A2]
Jump backward with feet together [A3 and A4]
Jump out with both feet to shoulder-width distance [A5]
Bring both feet together again [A6]
Bend your arms [A7]
Straighten your arms and execute one push-up [A8]
Jump forward with both feet [A9]
Straighten your knees and return to the starting position [A10]

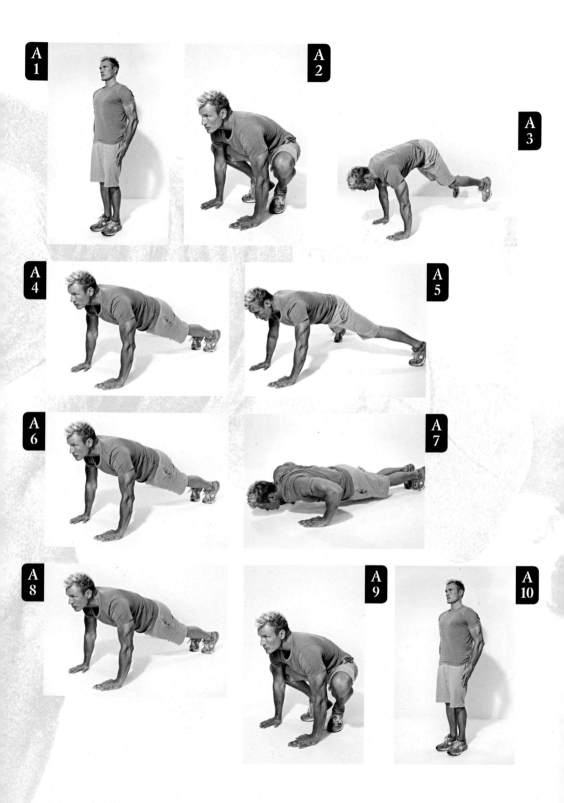

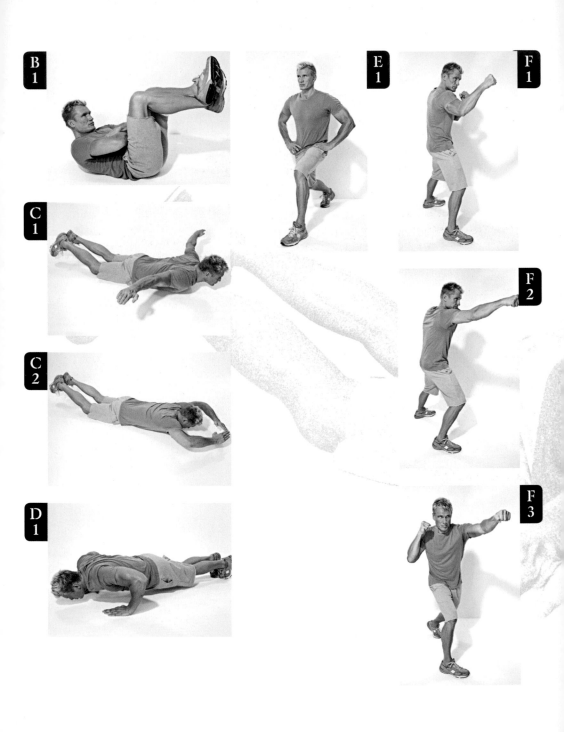

TRAINING BLOCK

Crunches (20 times)

Lie on your back with your knees bent, legs at a 90-degree angle. Keep your hands behind your neck or in front of your chest. Roll up your upper body, hold the top position for half a second, and then return slowly to the starting position [B1].

Back flyes (20 times)

Lie on your stomach, stretch your arms out to the sides like wings and lift your legs and head off the floor [C1]. With straight arms, bring your hands forward until they are in front of your face [C2] and keeping your legs and head above the floor, return your arms to the original wing position. Repeat.

Push-ups (20 times)

Perform push-ups on your hands or knuckles [D1].

Lunges (20 times per leg)

Keeping your hands on your hips, your eyes straight ahead, step forward with one leg into a lunge position [E1]. Lunge out with the other leg. That's one repetition.

Punching Combination (10 times per leg)

Assume a fighting position with your right leg forward and your clenched fists protecting your face [F1]. Punch straight out with the right knuckles [F2] and then follow up with a left punch [F3]. Return to the guard position. Switch to left leg forward after 10 punch combinations.

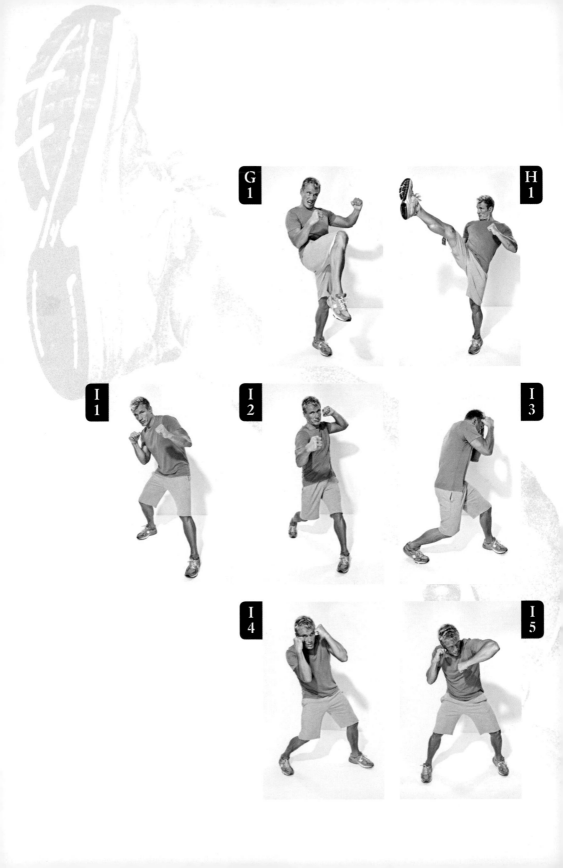

TRAINING BLOCK
Karate knee kick (10 times per leg)
Stand with your left leg forward with your fists in front of your face. Pull the right knee upward/forward then return to the starting position [G1]. Repeat. Switch legs after 10 knee kicks.

Front Kick (10 times per leg)
Stand with your left leg forward and a guard in front of your face. Lift your knee and kick out with your foot straight for the opponent's the solar plexus [H1]. Do not fully extend your leg. This takes stress off the knee joint. Repeat. Switch legs after 10 kicks.

Shadowboxing (30 seconds)
Assume a fighting position with your fists in front of your face and one leg in front [I1]. Shadow box, moving lightly on the balls of your feet, shifting your upper body and head from side to side [I3 and I4]. Use the jab, straight cross, and hooks [I2 and I5]. Add knee kicks and straight front kicks. Try rotating to the right and left, while throwing combinations.

TRAINING BLOCK

Leg Lifts (20 times)
Lie on your back with your hands under your lower back. Lift your legs up and down, with your knees slightly bent. Start from 2 inches above the floor and lift up to a 45-degree angle [J2].

Static back exercise (20 seconds)
Lie on your stomach, hands out to your sides, and hold this position while you count slowly to twenty [K1].

Everest push-ups (20 times)
Place your hands on the floor so that your body is bent at a 45-degree angle [L1]. Keep your hands shoulder-width apart and do a push-up [L2], returning to the "Everest" position. This works the shoulders and upper part of the chest.

Squats (20 times)
Stand with your feet shoulder-width apart and your hands in front of your chest. Bend your knees to a position just before 90 degrees [M1] and then straighten up again. You can set a chair behind you to make sure you hit the same down position each time. Let your buttocks touch the seat of the chair.

"Half-chins" (10 times)
Use a towel to protect your hands and take a shoulder-width grip on the upper side of a door. Don't worry, the load on the hinges isn't as great as you think, but try it slowly just to be sure. Lift yourself up to the door's top then lower yourself slowly until your arms are at a 90-degree angle. Pull yourself up again [N1]. Repeat.

Shadowboxing (1 minute)
Stand in front of a mirror or open window and shadow box for one minute.

Stop and unwind with the **DL stretch** (see page 110).

Total time for DL No Excuses: 15 minutes

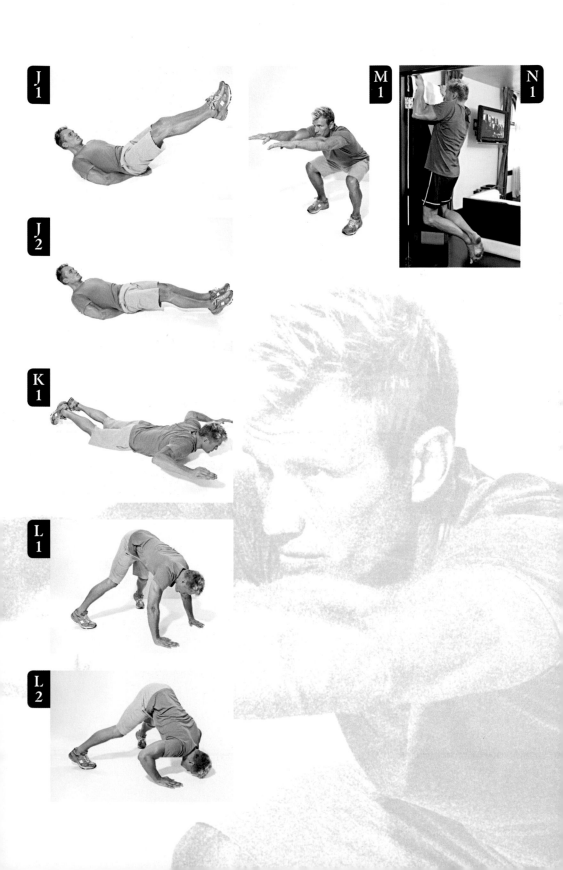

J
1

J
2

K
1

L
1

L
2

M
1

N
1

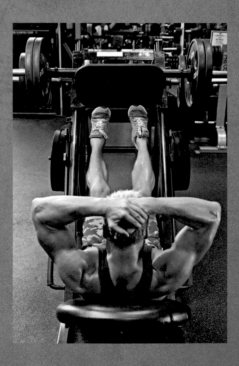

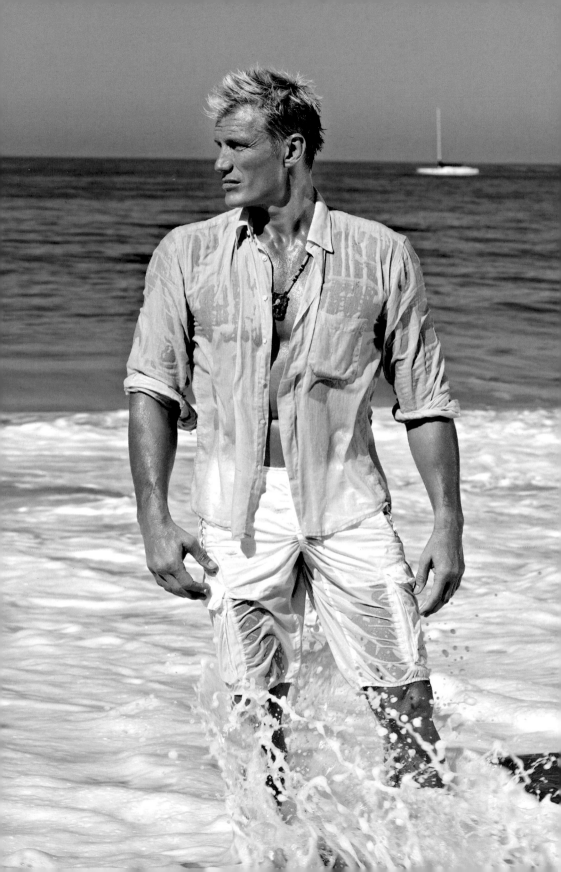

I was continuing my engineering studies in Sydney, Australia. My new girlfriend, singer Grace Jones, was back home in the United States. We had some phone contact, but were busy with our respective lives on different continents. In the eighties you had to order an "international operator assisted call" and stay on the line at least 10–15 minutes while an operator connected the call. No iPhones in those days.

I finally graduated from University of Sydney. Since the academic year in the southern hemisphere is one term "ahead" of the American school I had applied to, I had a gap of six months before it was time to go to the United States for further study. I had graduated number one in my class and gained admission into my dad's favorite school: MIT in Boston.

I decided to go to Japan to train with Mas Oyama, the great karate Master and the creator of the Kyokushin style of karate. Coincidentally, this worked out perfectly for Grace, too, because she was also going to Japan to do a TV commercial.

I went to Japan and trained seriously as I had intended, but I also took the opportunity to spend more time with Grace. Now we had more time for each other and started to fall in love for real. We talked about the near future. She invited me back to the United States. I would be studying in Boston soon and New York City, where she lived, was sort of on the way. As part of my engineering degree, I needed to do some practical work in a technical industry. I decided on New York.

Once I had got myself situated in the "Big Apple," some of Grace's friends in the fashion industry said that I should work as a male model. I followed their advice and did a number of photo shoots and earned extra money. When I wasn't taking pictures, I trained hard. My workout routine was still just as serious, both in the weight room and the karate dojo. With my height, Scandinavian looks, and athlete's physique, I stood apart from the average model in those days. Many male fashion photographers opened the door, swallowed hard, and began the audition with: "Okay, start by taking your shirt off."

Often, I got comments from friends like, "You look like you should be in the movies. You have muscles. You can fight. There has to be something you can do in Hollywood." I started to wonder: was it possible to make it as an actor?

This still seemed like a crazy idea to me. When the people around me kept pushing, I became more curious. Guess I've always found it difficult to walk away from a challenge. Here was a new one: the thought of a career in the movies had been planted in me. It sounded just crazy enough to be worth a try.

When it was time to start at MIT, I headed up to Boston to get set up. I'd planned to stay in Boston for at least a year, probably more. But my mind had already started to veer off in a different direction. After my experiences in Manhattan, further scientific pursuits just didn't seem that exciting. It was absurd: I had worked my ass off to get into one of the world's most respected schools. Now I found it hard to motivate myself toward further engineering studies.

In Manhattan, next to Grace, Andy Warhol, and others, I had experienced a world of creativity that seemed more alluring than anything I'd known before. The professors in the Chemical Engineering department probably thought the same as they stared out the window and saw a black motorcycle glide by. Driven by a blond giant in a leather jacket with an equally leather-clad Grace Jones on the back.

I didn't care that MIT was Dad's favorite school. After two weeks I went back to New York and my studies in Boston were replaced by acting classes in Manhattan. It went well and was much more fun than I had hoped for. When I was younger and suffered from allergies, I painted with oils, played music, and clowned around on the high school stage, even though I felt shy inside. Now I finally got to live this out. It was a huge boost to express an inner creativity that I had brushed aside in my adult life. I was actually was told by my acting coach that I had talent. He said that I was an emotional person. That the reason I had tried these different things in life was I was "a frustrated artist." Could he be right? How could I take advantage of that ability?

I knew that the competition for parts in the film and television industry was fierce, but it didn't matter. I enjoyed the excitement of putting up new scenes in acting class on a regular basis. I had yet to come face-to-face with a large audience or the lens of a movie camera.

As was my habit, I continued with karate training. I knew that it was soon time for the World

Championship in Kyokushin Karate, but I had no plans to compete. On the contrary, I had already made a decision to break away from fighting. How could I do that now, when I had my sights set on becoming the next Marlon Brando?

I was an accomplished fighter—one of the top ten in the Kyokushin karate world at that time. Now, prominent figures in that sport tried to find me. They definitely wanted me to have a crack at the World Championships in Tokyo later that year. It was just that nobody really knew where to find me.

They knew I had been fighting when I was studying in Australia, but the trail stopped there. Not many people knew that I had shipped off to the United States with Grace Jones. Remember, this was way before e-mail and Facebook. Even fewer people knew that I had put college on hold, what I was doing in New York, or that I was even there. Not even my parents.

I was later told that phones and faxes went hot between Sweden and Japan trying to locate me: "We want Lundgren to fight. But where do we find him?" Both Master Mas Oyama in Japan and my coach Brian Fitkin in Sweden were looking high and low. They finally tracked me down and insisted that I fight at the World Championships, only to be met by the answer, "Sorry, I can't help you. I'm a little busy over here."

And so it was that karate disappeared from my world for quite a number of years.

I continued with my acting classes, got a work visa to the US as a model. I somehow couldn't reveal to my family that I had dropped out of my Fulbright Scholarship at MIT to become a starving actor.

"So how are your studies going?" my father would ask over the phone. I could, without lying, simply say "Just great!" since I was still studying acting. I had

also gotten a microscopic supporting role in a Bond film with Grace. However, I had also begun to appear with her at various nightclubs in Manhattan. Somebody in the Swedish press got the clue: "Isn't he Swedish?"

A few weeks later, my dad came home after work had his coffee and opened the evening paper. There was a gossip article about "Grace Jones's new 'boy toy,'" with a picture of his son, the engineering student. "Who the hell is Grace Jones?"

A few days later, he turned on the TV and there was a black woman in a crew cut wearing a men's suit marching across stage singing "Demolition Man!" He noticed the artist's name: Grace Jones.

It was obvious that his son had lost his mind. ◐

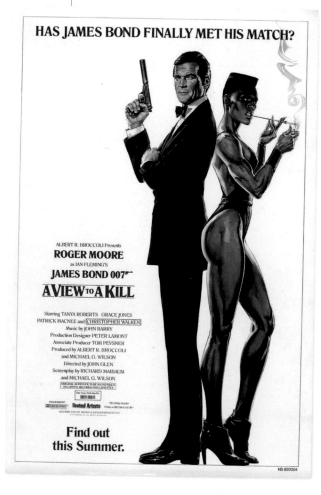

HAS JAMES BOND FINALLY MET HIS MATCH?

ALBERT R. BROCCOLI Presents
ROGER MOORE
as IAN FLEMING'S
JAMES BOND 007™
A VIEW TO A KILL

Starring TANYA ROBERTS GRACE JONES
PATRICK MACNEE and CHRISTOPHER WALKEN
Music by JOHN BARRY
Production Designer PETER LAMONT
Associate Producer TOM PEVSNER
Produced by ALBERT R. BROCCOLI
and MICHAEL G. WILSON
Directed by JOHN GLEN
Screenplay by RICHARD MAIBAUM
and MICHAEL G. WILSON

United Artists

Find out
this Summer.

NS 850004

DL GOODNIGHT STRETCH

5 MINUTES

A relaxing, yoga-inspired stretching routine that helps you unwind and reduce the tension in your body. These movements open up the joints in the body and relax the muscles. It is important that you focus on breathing during these exercises. Breathe in through your nose for 2 seconds and out through your half-open mouth for 5 seconds.

The routine ends with lying on the floor, putting your feet up against a wall, which relaxes the lower back and feet/calves.

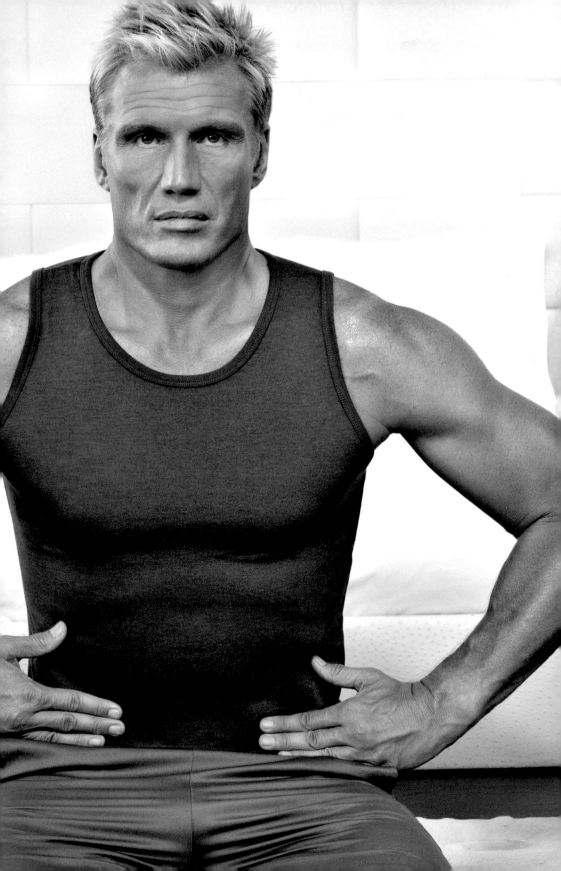

142

Seated isometric neck stretch (3 times)

Assume a seated position with your legs bent underneath you and lock your fingers behind your neck. Breathe in through your nose and gently pull with your hands to stretch the neck muscles forward/downward [A1]. Repeat.

"Wing stretch" (3 times)

Sit in the same position. Place the back of your hands against the upper part of your thighs [B1]. Stick your elbows out to the side and lean forward/downward. Breathe in and out three times while you stretch your back [B2].

Cat stretch (3 times)

Reach with your arms forward, shoulder-width apart and stretch your back for three deep breaths [C1].

Lumbar Stretch, lying down—left/right

Lie on the floor and stretch your lower back to the right and to the left [D1].

Relaxation with your feet against the wall—2 minutes

Put your feet up against a wall at a 45-degree angle. Relax and breathe slowly for 2 minutes [E1]. This helps to remove waste products from the legs and feet. This is a good time to mentally go through the next day's workout.

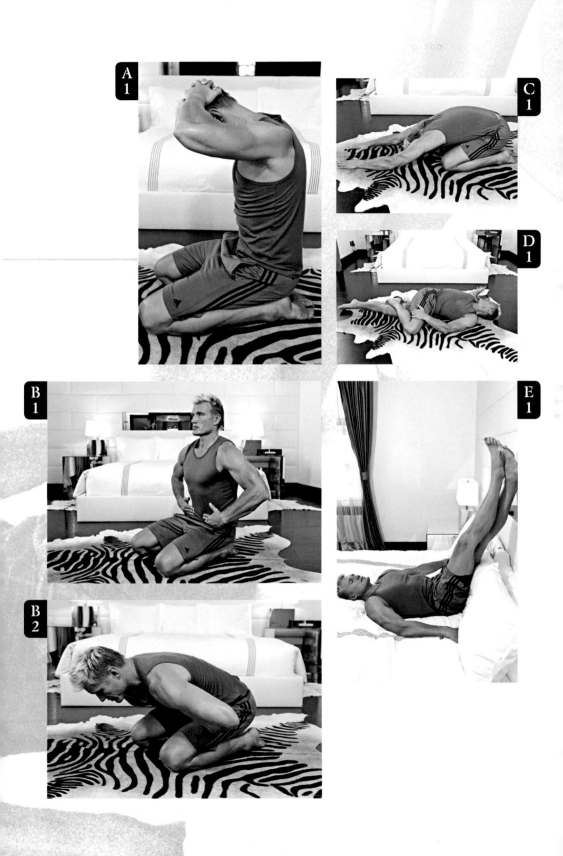

144

I kept fighting in New York, both at the gym and in my acting class. I did heavy weight training and had started to spend a good deal of time at one of the major boxing gyms in Manhattan: "Gleason's Gym."

I had a slightly different appearance than most of the fighters who trained there, to put it mildly. Nearly all the promising boxing talents were Hispanic or African-American. There seems to always be the same glimmer of opportunity that ignites in coaches and managers when they see a big white guy who can fight. Very rarely do they live up to expectations: throughout the twentieth century there have only been a handful of heavyweight champions who were Caucasian. My countryman Ingemar Johansson was the most recent and he won the title in 1959. Since then, many boxing managers have dreamt about signing the next "Great White Hope."

I was spotted straight away. Someone had studied me carefully during training and thought I moved extremely well for being so big . . . and white. I was approached with an offer to pursue a professional career as a boxer. Naturally, I was flattered by all the praise and was receptive to the idea.

I had great athletic confidence from my karate competitions. How far could I go in boxing? Dangerously empty of self-criticism, my ambitions started to run out of control.

It didn't seem too unreasonable that one day I would stand there in the middle of the ring with the heavyweight championship belt around my waist. I would be the immensely wealthy and famous new world heavyweight champion. "Easy!"

I accepted the offer to become a professional boxer. We went as far as to draw up a contract and it looked as if Mr. Lundgren would take another sharp turn in a highly unexpected direction in life.

The very day I was to sign the contract, I started to change my mind. I had fortunately listened to my friends, including Grace, who had joined forces against me. They finally convinced me that life as professional boxer was anything but a cakewalk.

Typically, a promising boxer gets to go maybe ten fights against some older burnt-out fighters, just to get some ring experience. Then if he is really lucky, he will get his chance against a top-ranked boxer. Lose that fight and it's goodbye career. There will never be another chance. Often it's goodbye physically too.

It wasn't like I could go back to studying at MIT after an unsuccessful professional boxing career.

Fortunately I came to my senses—while I still had them and my brain intact.

What I didn't know was that heavyweight boxing would change my life forever in a completely unexpected way. A few months later my agent in New York sent me on a casting call—"for some boxing movie."

Sly Stallone and Hollywood were waiting. ○

> I was hitting the heavy bag at Gleason's, when I heard someone approaching. Suddenly a teenage kid delivered a message: "He says he wants to kick your ass!" My eyes followed his pointed finger to a big black fighter at around the 240-lb mark who glared at me with a grim smile.
>
> There was a hard, no-nonsense attitude to these fighters. Many assumed that I got an offer for a professional boxing career only because of my looks, which was probably at least a little true.
>
> Many of the bigger guys in the gym were waiting for the chance to get up in the ring and kick my ass. I had some good sparring sessions in that place.

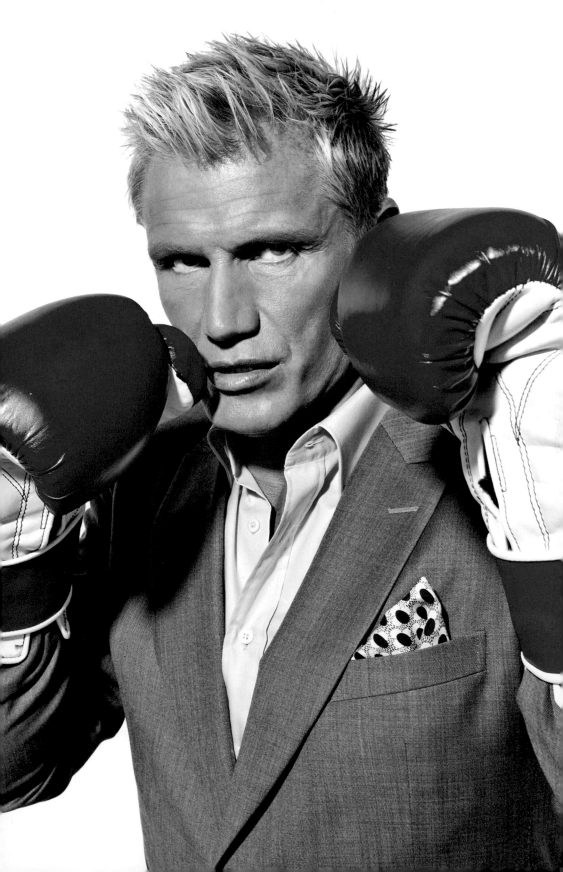

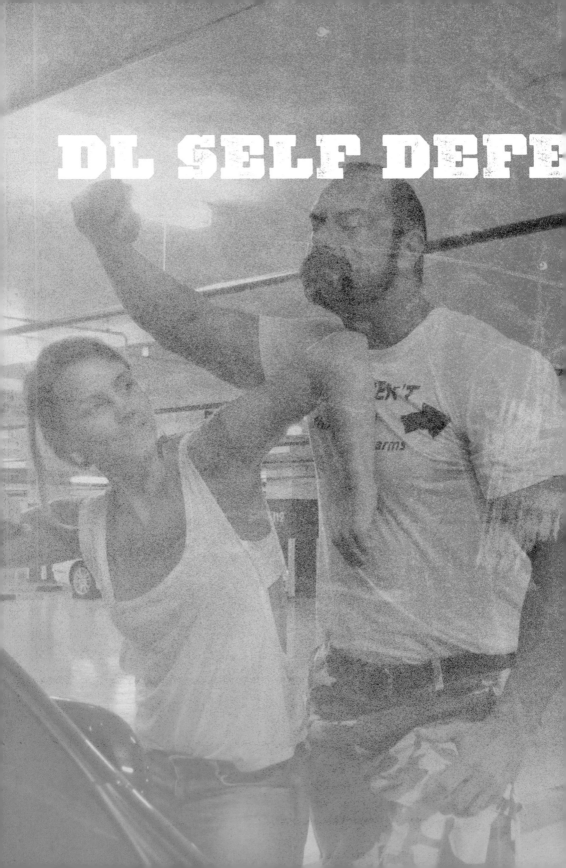

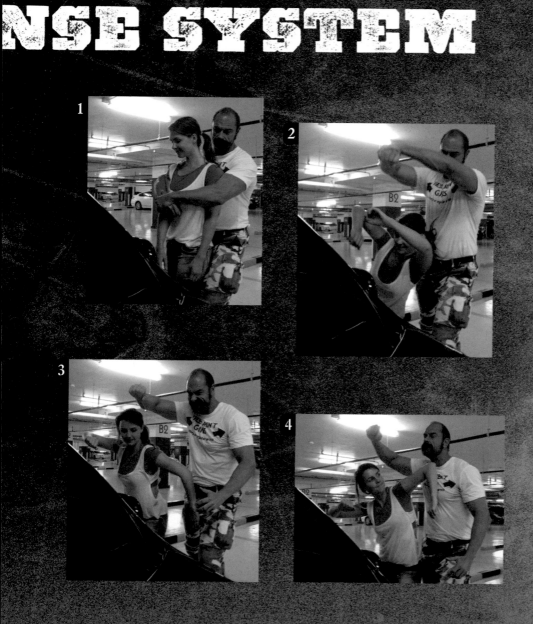

AGAINST GRAB FROM BEHIND

Drop straight down [2].
Strike backward with the hand to the groin [3].
Strike upward with an elbow to the chin [4].

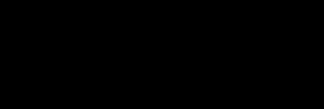

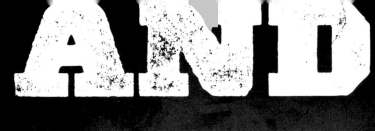

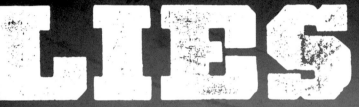

ARE YOU WHAT YOU EAT?

Make sure that your nutritional habits support your training. Stick to a few basic rules and be consistent. Eating right should be enjoyable.

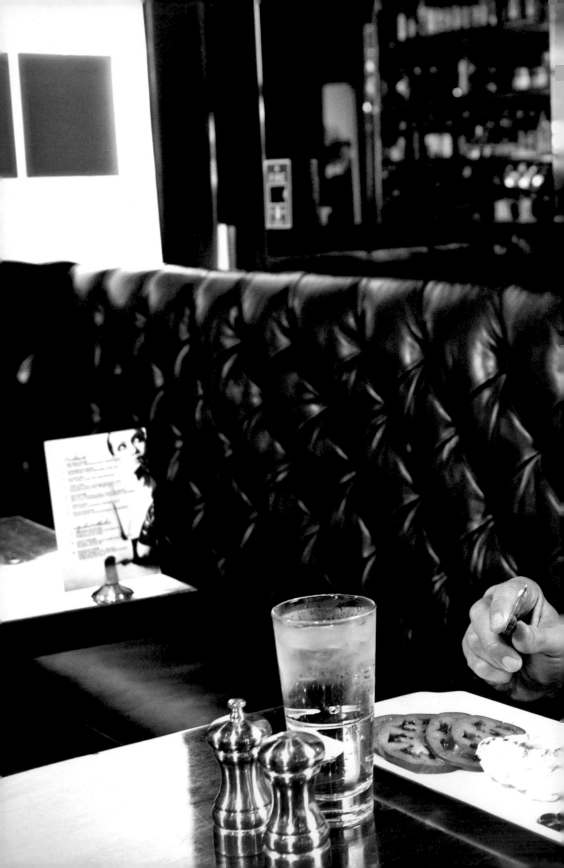

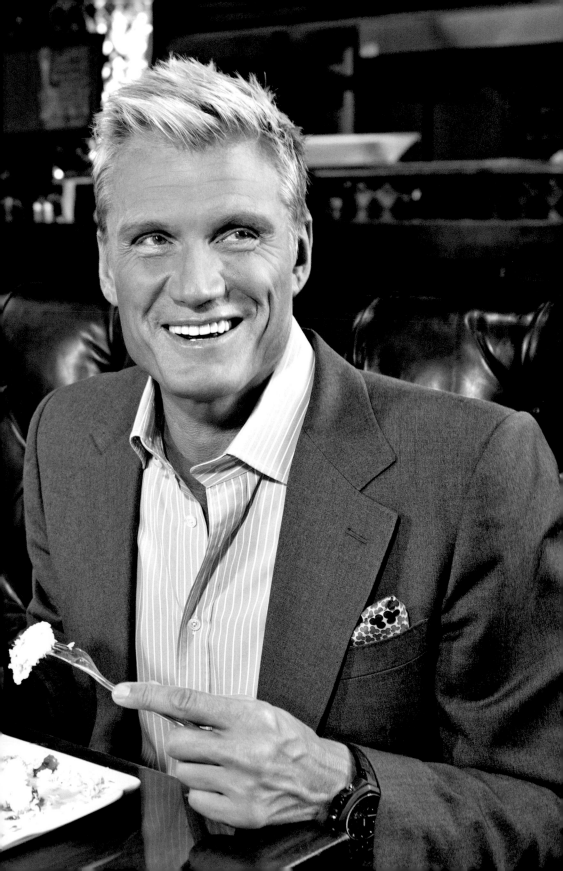

152

You can't write a book about training without getting into the complex field of diet and nutrition. The subject is vast and there are countless experts who have written heaps of literature on it. Yours truly is primarily interested in the practical applications, but my master's degree in Chemical Engineering gives me a chance to understand the physiological basis of nutrition.

For three decades, I have tested and evaluated most kind of nutritional advice there is.

I usually had specific goals in mind, such as preparing for various film roles or demanding karate competitions.

It is based on this experience I'd like to give you my thoughts on how to eat right.

FORGET THE "CRASH DIETS"

Sure, you can achieve short-term weight loss or gain by adhering to a strict diet for a few weeks. But it's not sustainable in the long run and it is definitely not healthy for your body. Remember, it's not about diet. It's about lifestyle. Any nutritional plan you go with has to work anytime, anywhere.

Dolph's three nutritional rules
1. Keep your blood sugar level constant
2. Eat a good breakfast
3. Remember protein

Blood sugar
When you wake up, your blood sugar levels are in the low range. When you eat a meal, the levels increase and after an hour or so they start to drop back to a "normal" range. Your goal should be keeping blood sugar levels in your normal range, i.e. don't eat too much sugar or starve yourself during the day. When your blood sugar is neither too high nor too low, your body burns calories effectively and you always feel alert. Keeping your blood sugar in that normal range also prevents your body from going into what's called "starvation mode," storing excess calories as fat. When your blood sugar is in the normal range, you feel both mentally sharp and physically alert. In practical terms this means that you should eat something every three or four hours while you are awake.

I usually try to imagine a chart in my mind. When I see that blood sugar graph start heading down, when I feel sluggish, tired, irritable, or crave coffee and sweets, that's when it's time to eat a real meal or have a healthy snack. More tips about this later.

Throughout my film career, I've had to maintain extreme diets for short periods of time. It's not something I recommend, but on some occasions I have been forced to go to extremes to achieve the right body for the part.

One of the most bizarre examples was during a shoot in Africa.

We worked long hours in extreme heat in the Namibian desert. The local producers told us how important it was to fill up on fluids at all times. The problem was that in the heat, any excess fluid was going to make my muscles appear less defined in front of the cameras. I had to restrict my water intake to look good in some key shirtless scenes. I went so far as to hire a local assistant whose sole mission was to carry a notepad to keep track of my water consumption during the day.

Desperately thirsty, I constantly begged for more water. He usually refused. When he was hired, I had told the guy, "Whatever I tell you, DON'T give me more than 2 fl. oz. water per hour, or you'll be fired."

The poor guy did his job, even though we almost got into a fist fight when he refused to give me the extra drops I begged for. "What do you mean, I had 14 oz. today? You're lying. Give me another 2."

"Nope!"

Breakfast

Most overweight and underweight people have one thing in common: they don't eat a proper breakfast. For me, breakfast is absolutely the most important meal of the day. Whether I exercise before breakfast or later in the day, I need enough nutrients in my first meal. Or I risk falling into the vicious cycle of fatigue, too much sugar, and late dinners.

If you want to fully indulge in a meal, let it be breakfast. Here you can have everything: protein, fat, and carbohydrates. Ice cream! Go for it.

Protein

To maintain your muscle mass, you need to ingest about ½ gram of protein per pound of bodyweight per day. If you train extra hard you need more. In practical terms, when I see a menu or go food shopping, I automatically think protein. When I am at a restaurant or standing in the kitchen, my immediate thought is, "meat, fish, or chicken?" Then comes the carbohydrate decision, like "potatoes or rice?" How many carbs I eat per day depends on how hard I work out, but I always eat the same amount of protein. I weigh 220 lbs. So how much is 110 grams of protein? Two eggs and oatmeal at breakfast, a tuna salad at lunch, a protein bar for a snack, and a large chicken breast at dinner. That's about 110 grams.

"Fast" and "slow" carbohydrates

One theory says that people started to eat larger amounts of carbohydrates when we learned how to make bread from cultivated grains. That's when we started to "think clearer," inventing tools and making technological advances that improved our living conditions. Our human carb-fueled brains have ruled the world ever since.

We need carbohydrates to think clearly and to work hard, but with today's eating habits it's easy to consume too much.

I try to be aware of the amount of carbohydrates I take in. If I am in a period of karate training, I have to load up on more energy or I'll be drained after one workout. If I train with less intensity, I try hold back on the rice, potatoes, and pasta, especially in the evenings.

It's important to eat carbs from the right sources. Today there are many foods containing added sugars, leading to an increased rate of obesity and type 2 diabetes. Fortunately, these relationships have been increasingly documented, which has resulted in popular methods to "eat right." This includes the so-called "GI-method," which uses a Glycemic Index (GI) to rank carbohydrates based on how quickly they raise your blood sugar levels. If you ingest "fast" carbohydrates (foods or drinks with high levels of refined sugars), you'll create sharp increases in your blood sugar levels. The level of blood sugar controls the amount of insulin secreted to balance the sugar level. The higher the blood sugar, the more insulin your body pumps into the bloodstream to maintain a balance. This struggle can put a strain on the body and, in the worst cases, can cause type 2 diabetes.

DOLPH'S FAVORITE ENERGY SOURCES

Good sources of carbohydrates:
Oatmeal
Potatoes
Root Vegetables
Fruits
Rice
Whole-grain bread

Good sources of protein:
Eggs
Fish
Meat
Chicken
Turkey

Good fat sources:
Avocado
Fish oil (including capsule form)
Olive oil
Nuts

So again: it's important to help your body keep your blood sugar levels steady. This is is what the GI-method is all about. You do this by selecting the "slow" carbohydrate sources that don't raise blood sugar levels so drastically. Examples of slow carbohydrates are rice, grains, and potatoes. Fast carbs are bread, sweets, and most soft drinks.

How much energy do you need?

Your body needs a certain amount of energy to deal with the work it has to perform. Modern humans have the Stone Age human's physique and metabolism. However, most of us don't live a nomadic life, walking tens of miles a day to hunt game or to gather firewood. Just staying alive required a lot of energy back then.

Since we don't have the same energy expenditure as our ancestors, we need to think more about the balance between our physical activity and the amount of food we consume.

The type of food we eat has changed dramatically, especially in the industrialized countries. A Stone Age man woke up and peered out of his cave, realizing he had fairly limited options for feeding himself and his family. He could look for birds' eggs, pick fruit, hunt for meat, fish, or dig for root vegetables. There were no chips, cheesecake, tacos, pizza, toast, or drive-in burger joints. These modern "food inventions" have only been around for two generations or so. Although sometimes satisfying to consume, we're better off sticking to a "Stone Age diet" most of the time.

Where does energy come from?

The energy sources in the foods you eat come from protein, fat, and carbohydrates. Most people who exercise want to build muscle and reduce body fat. The type of food you eat plays a major role here.

How do I incorporate all this information into my diet in an easy way?

A simple rule: "Eat breakfast like a king, lunch like a prince, and dinner like a poor man!"

That rule works for me. I always try to load up at breakfast and scale back as the day goes on. You can "reset" your metabolism by having a full breakfast.

Once in a while I like to go out to a good restaurant to have a nice dinner. I love a medium-rare NY steak, slightly charred on the outside, and a fully loaded baked potato. Oh, and cheesecake for dessert. A good red wine perfects the meal. We all need it sometimes.

Nutrition is an individual thing and you have to get a feel for what works best for you.

Here are some examples of my favorite breakfasts, lunches, and dinners as inspiration. These meals are healthy and taste good, in my opinion!

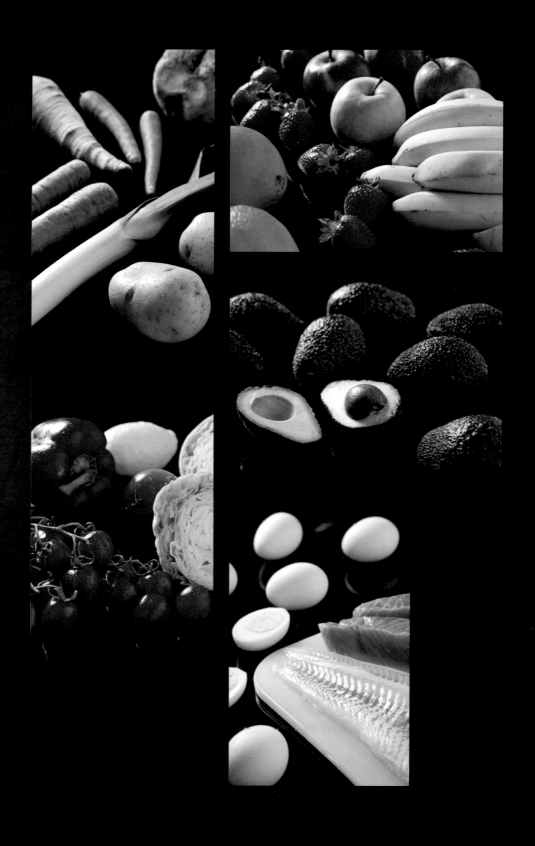

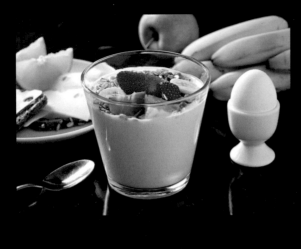
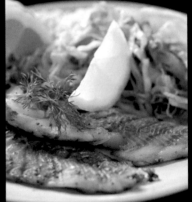
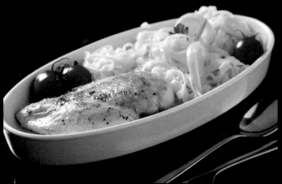
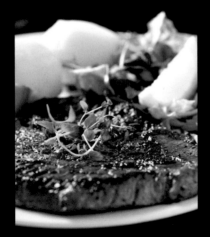
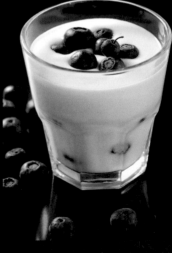

OPTIONS FOR A PERFECT FOOD DAY

Breakfast

1. Scrambled eggs—try mixing one egg and two egg whites. Fresh blueberries. Two slices of full-grain bread with honey and sliced cheese.
2. Oatmeal with sliced banana, honey, cinnamon, and skim milk. Two hard-boiled eggs with whole-grain toast.
3. Yogurt with muesli and mixed fruit. Two slices of whole-grain bread with honey or a bran muffin.
4. Protein shake—yogurt, a banana, blueberry, honey, 20 grams of whey protein, a raw egg, and a little ice.

If I'm going to do a hard workout, I'll opt for breakfast 1 or 2.

Mid-morning snack

1. Protein drink
2. A banana and a protein bar
3. Yogurt with fruit and honey

Lunch

1. Grilled fish with rice, a green salad
2. Caesar salad with grilled chicken breast
3. Cured salmon with potato salad
4. Meatballs with mashed potatoes
5. Pasta with chicken breast

Afternoon snack

1. An over-the-counter protein drink and a banana (especially if I'm going to train in the evening)
2. A green apple and a bag of peanuts

Dinner

1. A steak with baked potatoes and vegetables
2. A grilled chicken breast with wild rice and vegetables
3. A large bowl of chicken soup with a cheese sandwich (light dinner)
4. Yogurt with fresh berries and bananas (even lighter dinner)

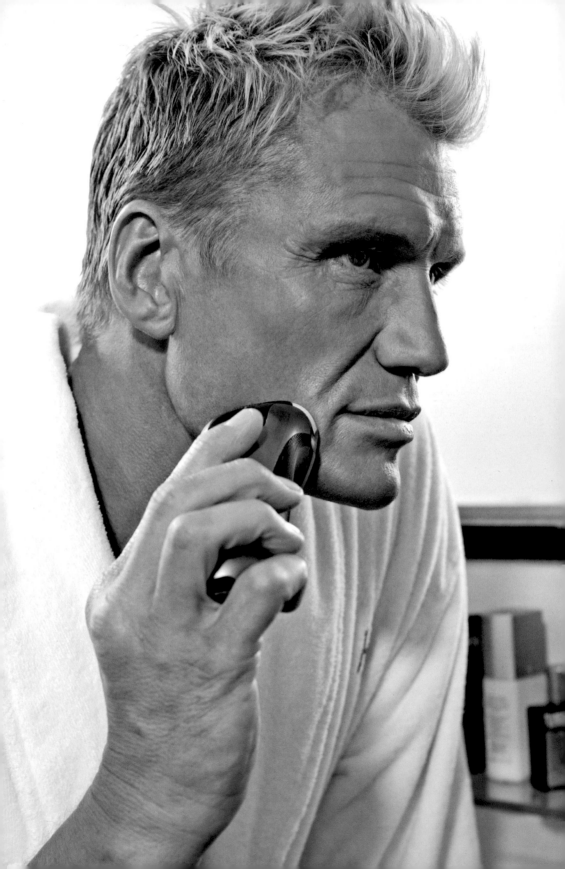

RECIPES FOR MY "DL SPECIALS"

DL Wake-up Shot
Half a glass of water
2 tbsp of MSM (methylsulfonylmethane in powder form. Helps with muscle soreness and joint pain.)
1 g of effervescent vitamin C (like a pack of Emergen-C)
3 tbsp of an energy drink (like 5-hour Energy or Red Bull)

Mix and drink first thing after you get up in the morning. This brew is especially effective if you're going to the gym before breakfast.

DL Muscle Shake
Low-fat yogurt
A banana
A raw egg
1 tbsp of honey
20 g of whey protein
3–4 ice cubes

Mix in a blender and serve after a workout, or for breakfast. Can also be made with cold water instead of yogurt. Peanut butter is another good ingredient you can add.

Regarding vitamins and supplements: this is very individual and the best way to approach this is to try out what your body responds to and needs. Here is my personal list:

Vitamins and supplements I take daily
One pack of multivitamins
1,000 mg of vitamin C in the morning with my Wake-up Shot.
1,500 mg glucosamine
2–3 g of MSM in the morning with my Wake-up Shot.
1,500 mg of omega-3 fish oil
20 g of whey protein in my Muscle Shake.

OCCASIONAL CHEATING IS FINE—AND ENJOYABLE

Sometimes you have to cheat on your nutritional commitments and enjoy what you crave: sweets, dessert, wine, a beer, or a cocktail, etc. Life is too short to always eat 100 percent healthy food. I tend to give myself special treats when I feel over-trained or when I'm under unusually difficult pressure from work.

After a tough karate session, it feels good to order a hamburger with French fries and have cheesecake for dessert. I like a good red wine with a steak. When I go back to Sweden there is nothing better than to head down to the corner and order a hot dog and a Coke. If you have too many low fat and "diet" foods your body's metabolism can begin to slow down. Your muscle recovery may suffer and you'll get nowhere with your workouts. Psychologically, it is also nice to be able to indulge in what you want. Why else do we train, if not to fully enjoy our lives?

For example, I like an Italian liqueur called Fernet Branca. Perfect as a digestive after dinner!

Coffee is another one of my favorite vices. There's nothing like a perfect double espresso macchiato with hot milk. If you just keep your coffee drinking reasonably under control, you don't have to worry. Enjoy a cup of coffee when sitting down at the computer, before heading down to the gym, or before you take that early morning walk.

I don't drink coffee after 5 p.m. It can affect your sleep. If I train in the evening, I prefer a protein shake or a banana for some extra energy.

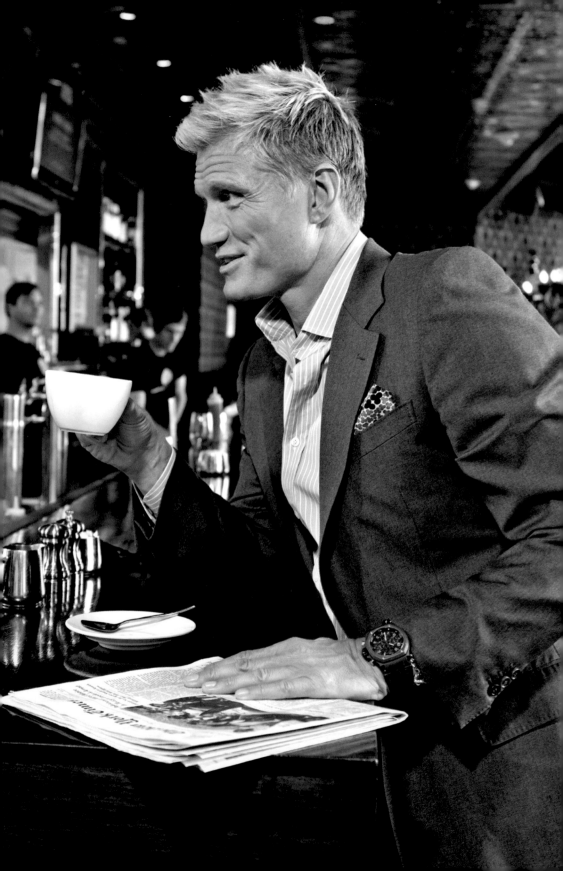

COMBINING FOOD WITH YOUR TRAINING PROGRAMS

Here are some examples of how I plan my nutritional intake during a typical training day. You will find detailed descriptions of the various training programs in Chapter 6, Tactics.

No Time
First thing in the morning: DL Wakeup Shot
No Excuses: 15 minute home exercise.
Breakfast: combine two egg whites and one whole egg into an omelet, a cup of
blueberries, two slices of whole wheat toast with honey, hot tea, apple juice
Snack 1: DL Muscle Shake
Lunch: tuna salad, fruit salad
Snack 2: a banana, cashew nuts
Dinner: grilled chicken breast with rice and vegetables
DL Goodnight stretch
Bedtime: hot chamomile tea with the juice of one lemon

Cruise
First thing in the morning: DL Wakeup Shot
DL stretch
Breakfast: oatmeal, a hard-boiled egg, juice, tea
Mid-morning: a cup of coffee
DL Program 4
Snack 1: DL Muscle Shake
Lunch: Caesar salad with chicken breast, fruit salad
Snack 2: one protein bar
Dinner: steak with salad and vegetables
DL Goodnight stretch
Bedtime: hot chamomile tea with lemon

Action star
First thing in the morning: DL Wakeup Shot
DL stretch
Breakfast: DL Muscle Shake
Snack 1: one banana
Lunch: grilled fish with potatoes and vegetables
Snack 2: a protein bar and nuts
DL Program 1
Dinner: Thai chicken soup with rice, fruit salad for dessert
DL Goodnight stretch
Bedtime: hot mint tea with lemon

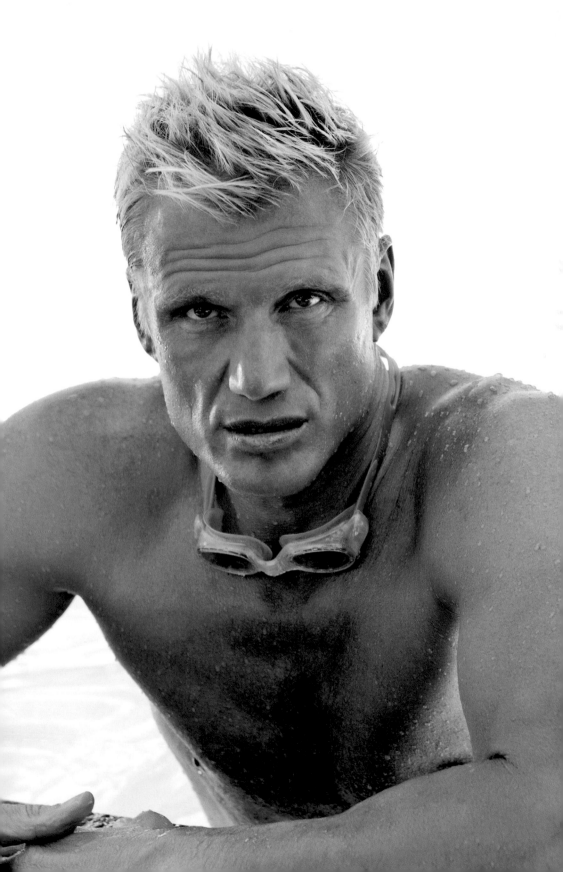

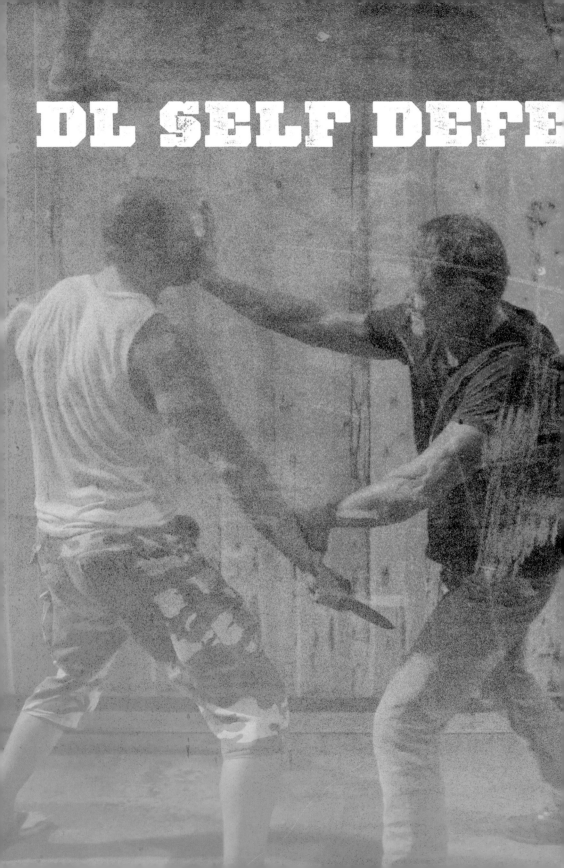

DL SELF DEFE

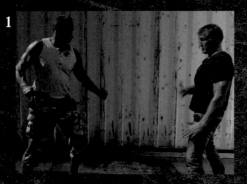

AGAINST A STRAIGHT KNIFE THRUST

Step back and parry in a circular motion
with your palm, keeping control of the knife [2].
Palm heel strike to the face [3].
Grab your opponent's head with the same hand
and execute a knee strike to the face [4].

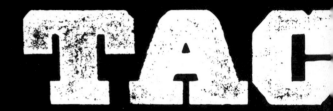

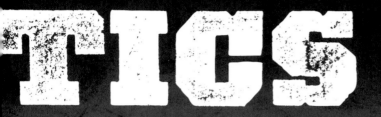

TICS

CREATE YOUR OWN BODY PLAN

You have decided to get in shape. You feel that you have the motivation and the proper tools. You understand that you have to give your body the right fuel. You need an overall plan. I'll show you how to use the workouts you've read about in this book. How you can create your own "body-plan." Further down, I'll explain how I prepared for *Rocky IV* and *The Expendables*.

SIX PROGRAMS FOR SUCCESS

In this chapter, I have put together a number of programs for a weekly training plan. With the right "tactics" you can be a winner.

All programs are composed of the workout routines described in Chapter 3, Weaponry, and Chapter 4, Special Ops. See these chapters for correct movements and the numbers of sets and reps to use.

Each program describes one week of training. A week is pretty easy to plan for, even when you're traveling or working hard at the office. You can use one program for a couple of weeks then move on to another program, depending on your progress and your practical situation.

For those who seek a more long-term commitment, I recommend my DL Body Plan. It uses all five programs over a period of eight weeks, easing you in with a soft start then gradually increasing to a serious effort.

Good luck!

1: NO TIME

Based entirely on working without equipment, you can do these sessions anytime, anywhere.
In addition to muscular strength you also improve your agility, coordination, and endurance.

Day 1: DL No Excuses
Day 2: DL No Excuses
Day 3: DL No Excuses
Day 4: 45 minutes cardio (cycling, cross country skiing, swimming, running, karate, etc.)

I use the No Time program when I travel a lot or want to take a break from the gym. It works well when you're back after the holidays, before moving on to harder training. It is perfect for those who have given up on exercise and want to start again!

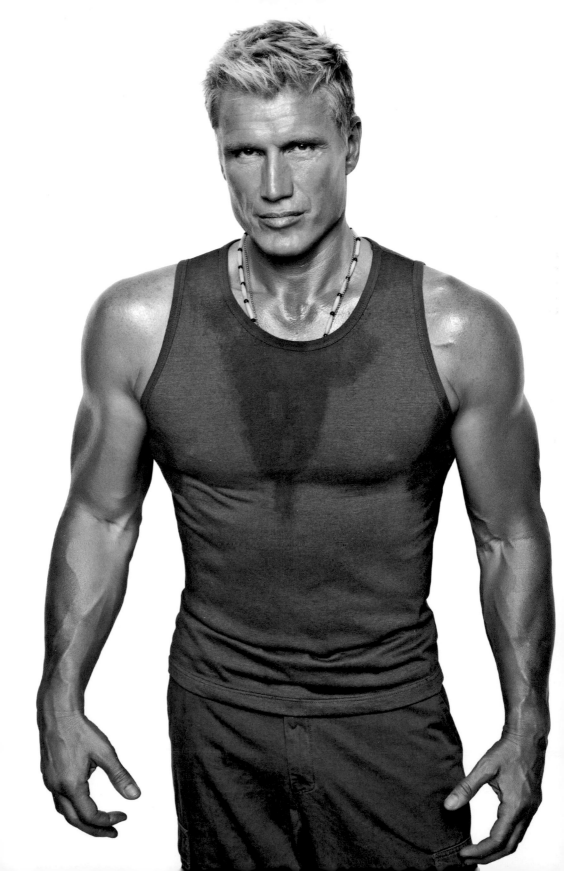

2: CRUISE

Combine the No Excuses exercises with circuit training with weights,
DL Program 4.

Day 1: DL No Excuses
Day 2: DL No Excuses
Day 3: DL No Excuses
Day 4: DL Program 4

Cruise is perfect if you find a decent hotel gym or want to shift into second gear
after a vacation.

3: MUSCLE UP

Muscle Up is my basic strength program to build muscle, based on progressive
training with weights. All muscle groups of your body are covered in three days.

Day 1: DL Program 1
Day 2: DL Program 2
Day 3: DL Program 3

If you work hard at the gym, remember that you need the rest to put on muscle.
Start easy, gradually increasing the weights you use.
Muscle Up is perfect for a longer period of results-oriented training.

4: LEAN AND MEAN

Lean and Mean adds a session of pure cardio each week. What type of cardio you
do is up to you. Everything from skiing to swimming or running will do the job.

Day 1: DL Program 1
Day 2: DL Program 2
Day 3: DL Program 3
Day 4: Cardio 45 minutes

Do cardio on a day when you don't lift weights, for example on the weekend. The
idea is to get a cross-training effect. Your body has to work both fast and slow-
twitch muscle fibers by combining strength and cardio sessions.

5: ACTION STAR

The Action Star is the foundation of my personal training. I do strength work for the entire body over three days, adding two cardio sessions of at least forty-five minutes each time.

The sixth session is either DL Program 4 with weights or a third cardio session, depending on how you feel that week and what works in practice. Remember, you need good sleep and nutrition to recover from these more demanding workouts.

Day 1: DL Program 1
Day 2: Cardio 45 minutes
Day 3: DL Program 2
Day 4: Cardio 45 minutes
Day 5: DL Program 3
Day 6: DL Program 4 or Cardio 45 minutes

I use Action Star to prepare for physically demanding film projects in Hollywood. My cardio is usually karate, boxing, or swimming.

6: DL BODY PLAN

For those who want a more detailed, long-term commitment, this is your program. It is a targeted training plan lasting eight weeks. Get your gym bag is packed and get ready to go!

The first week includes the home workout routines, the second week will take you further into the gym, and so on. Week by week the intensity increases gradually. The last week, you'll do all four weight training sessions and two cardio sessions for a full Action Star week. This should give you the results you want.

Week 1: No Time Program
Week 2: Cruise Program
Week 3: Cruise Program
Week 4: Muscle Up Program
Week 5: Muscle Up Program
Week 6: Lean and Mean Program
Week 7: Lean and Mean Program
Week 8: Action Star Program

Always remember: Stretch for 5 minutes after every hard workout. Eating right and sleeping are just as important as exercise. If you are sick or injured: SKIP A SESSION!

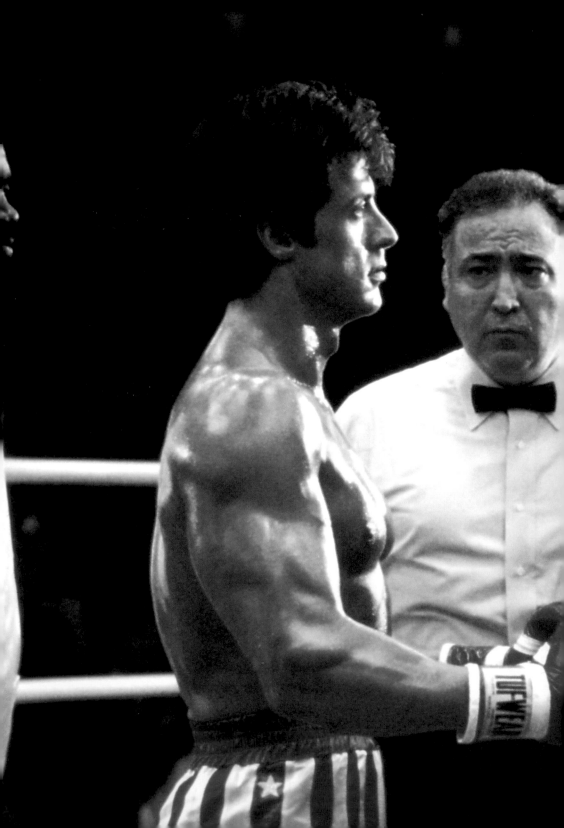

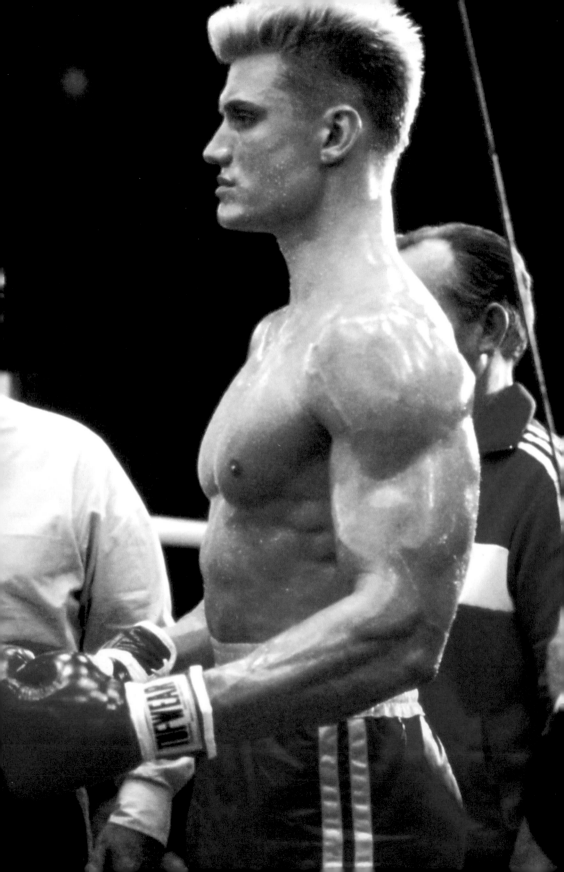

ROCKY IV

For my role in *Rocky IV*, Sly Stallone and I used a combination of boxing and weight training to achieve the professional boxer's muscular, athletic physique. There were many scenes where we not only had to look right, but had to perform the physically grueling boxing sequences and training montages. No computer special effects in those days. It all had to be real.

For six months, I prepared for my screen test with a workout program that was very similar to Action Star on page 171—weight training four times a week combined with cardio.

After getting the role and moving from New York to Los Angeles, Sly and I got down to some serious training. We trained six days a week for five months— weights for an hour in the morning and two hours of boxing in the afternoon.

It looked something like this:

Monday: chest/back in the morning and boxing in the afternoon
Tuesday: shoulders/arms in the morning and boxing in the afternoon
Wednesday: legs in the morning and boxing in the afternoon
Thursday: chest/back in the morning and boxing in the afternoon
Friday: shoulders/arms in the morning and boxing in the afternoon
Saturday: legs in the morning and boxing in the afternoon
Sunday: rest

We basically used a classic three-day "split" program for the whole body, plus the boxing for cardio. After five months of getting in super shape with this program, Stallone remarked: ". . . now it's impossible to get out of shape."

Pages 172-173: Rocky Balboa and Ivan Drago in *Rocky IV*

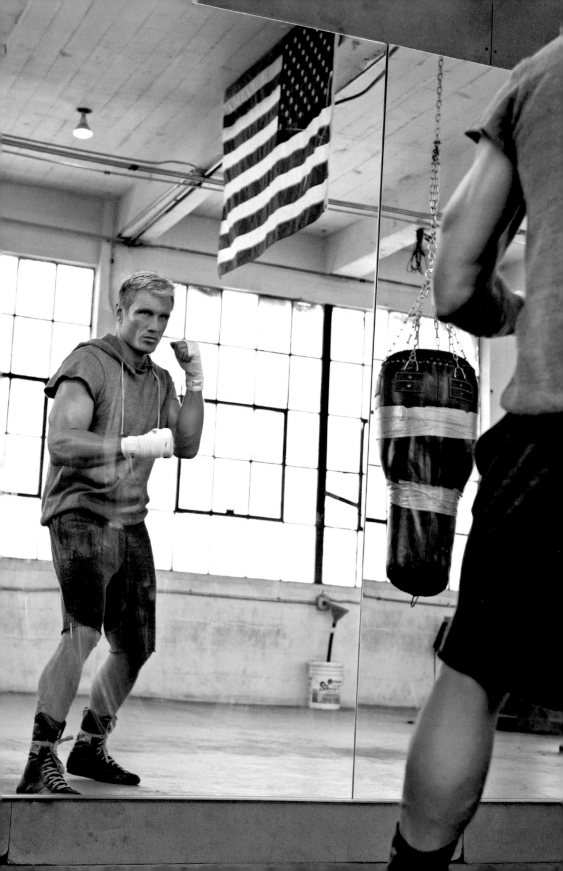

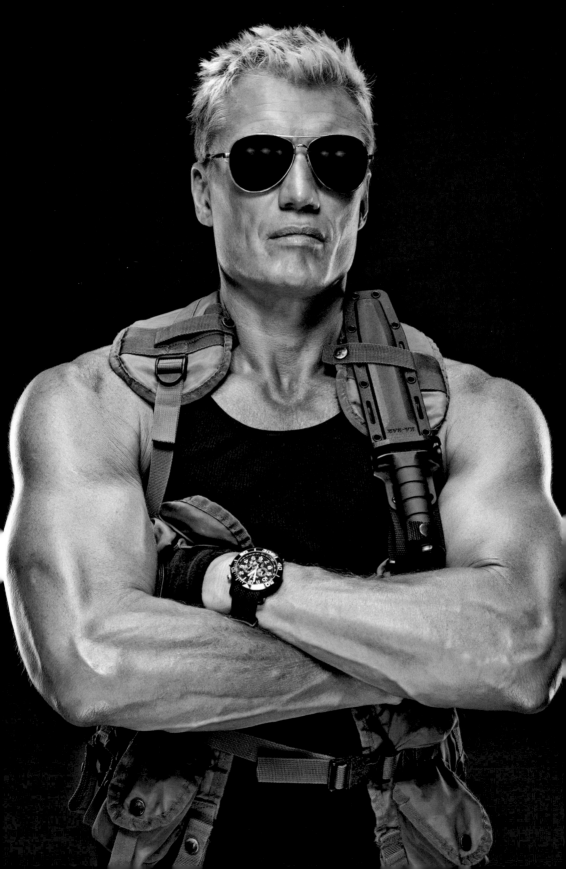

THE EXPENDABLES

In *The Expendables*, I knew would be sharing the screen with not only Sly Stallone, but huge guys like wrestler Steve Austin (250 lbs) and football player Terry Crews (240 lbs). So I decided to ease back on the legs, chest, and back workouts. Instead, I focused on my shoulders and arms three days a week with a special "reverse pyramid" program with dumbbells.

Warm up using light dumbbells. Then start your first set with heavy dumbbells, decreasing the weight while increasing the number of repetitions as you go through the sets. This is the reverse of a traditional "pyramid" workout. No rest between sets. Rest for 2 minutes between exercises.

1. "Arnold" dumbbell press (see page 75)
Warm up with 15 reps, then 6, 8, 10, 12 reps
Rest
2. Combination shoulder exercise (see page 75)
Warm up with 12 reps, then 4, 6, 8, 10 reps
Rest
3. Standing biceps curl (see page 76)
Warm up with 12 reps, then 4, 6, 8, 10 reps
Rest
4. Concentration curl (see page 76)
Warm up with 15 reps, then 6, 8, 10, 12 reps
Rest
5. Lying triceps press (see page 76)
Warm up with 15 reps, then 6, 8, 10, 12 reps
Rest
6. Forearm curl behind the back (see page 66)
Warm up with 15 reps, then 6, 8, 10, 12 reps

You'll get a great pump and be ready to show off your "guns" in a cut-off *Expendables* T-shirt!

Page 178: Dolph and Terry Crews

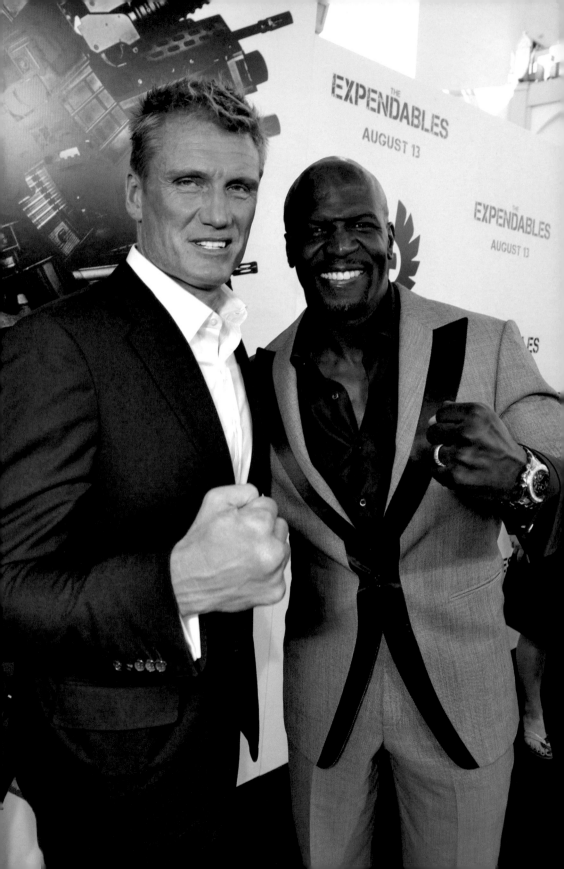

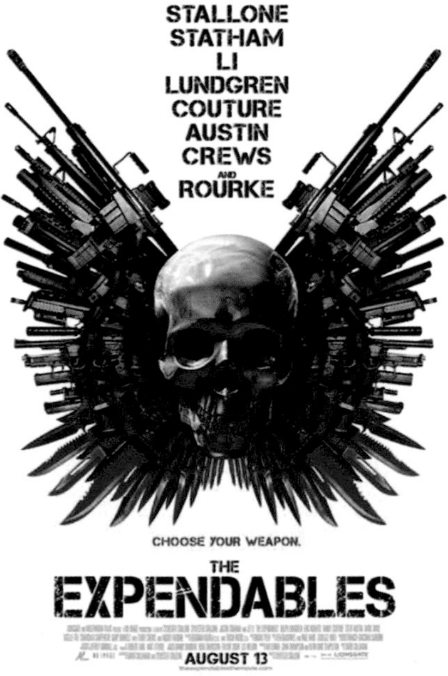
STALLONE
STATHAM
LI
LUNDGREN
COUTURE
AUSTIN
CREWS
AND
ROURKE
CHOOSE YOUR WEAPON.
THE
EXPENDABLES
AUGUST 13

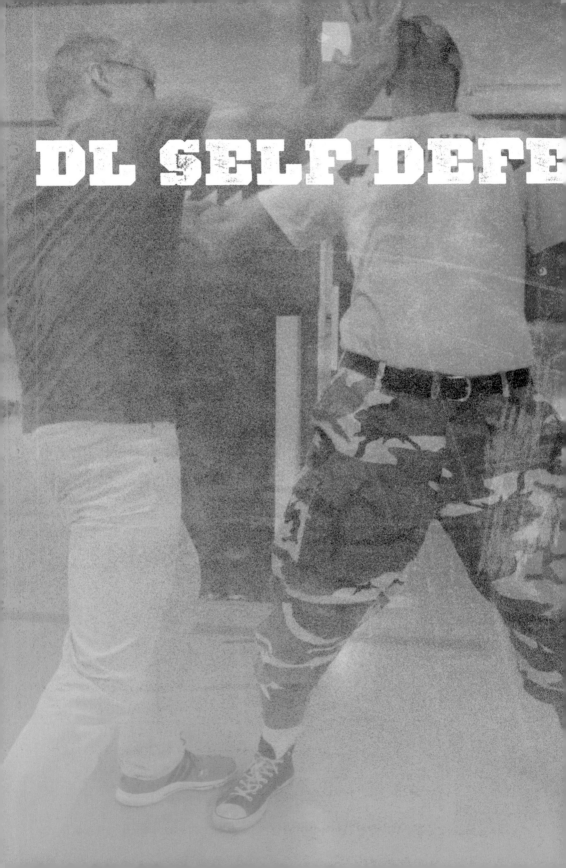

NSE SYSTEM

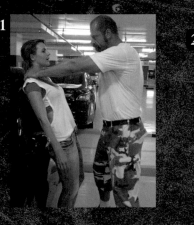

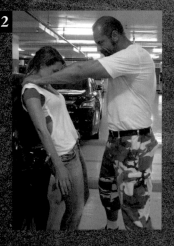

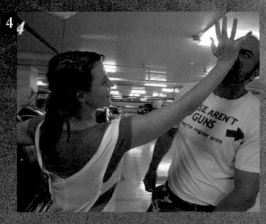

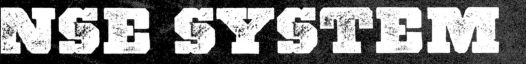

AGAINST A FRONTAL STRANGLE HOLD

Tuck in your chin to prevent the assailant from
crushing your wind pipe [2].
Knee to the groin [3].
Follow up with a palm heel strike to the nose [4].

So how did the story end for the shy Swedish kid who left for Hollywood to appear in that "boxing movie"? He became better known as actor Dolph Lundgren, making some fifty films over thirty years.

Grace and I went our separate ways after *Rocky IV* premiered, but are still friends.

After a break, I continued practicing karate with my mentor Brian Fitkin and I'm always a welcome guest at his dojo in Stockholm. As with most actors, my film career has gone up and down. Right now it is sort of up because of the action-franchise *The Expendables* with my original sparring-partner Sylvester Stallone, Arnold Schwarzenegger, and the rest of the action gang. *The Expendables 3* is being released this fall. I trained hard for these films.

The actor also became a director and I am preparing for my sixth directing project, which I also wrote. I just wrapped a picture that I wrote, produced, and starred in called *Skin Trade*, dealing with human trafficking. My master's degree was perhaps not entirely wasted after all.

> SO, MY FRIENDS, I SEE NO OTHER OPTION THAN TO PACK MY GYM BAG, DOWN A PROTEIN SHAKE, AND HEAD OVER TO THE GYM FOR A WORKOUT.

I think my father would be pleased. He died about ten years after I moved to Hollywood, but he got the chance to see his son achieve success and happiness. We became good friends in the end, even though we never could speak about what happened so long ago. I forgive him for all the bad things he did, because I know that deep down he loved me. **I thank him for the drive to go out into the world** and seek new challenges. For coming to Hollywood and making it as an actor. "A man's gotta do something for a living," to quote Clint Eastwood.

I have begun to feel more of my injuries from my fighting career and those fifty action movies. I have to deal with a bad ankle and an injured vertebra in my lower back. Sure, it's becoming a bit tougher to stay in shape, but I just have to dig in. I know that my body, as that of other strong and seemingly invulnerable men before me, will eventually be reduced to dust. I feel a sense of awe when I think back to all of the physical feats I've been involved in on various film sets, in the dojo, and in the gym. It's amazing what the human body can handle when you decide to push yourself.

We must all find our path to a fulfilling life. All through history, men have had the same feelings as you and I have toward the brief and transient nature of our earthly existence.

So, my friends, I see no other option than to pack my gym bag, down a protein shake, and head over to the gym for a workout.

Training is my life.

I wouldn't have it any other way. ○

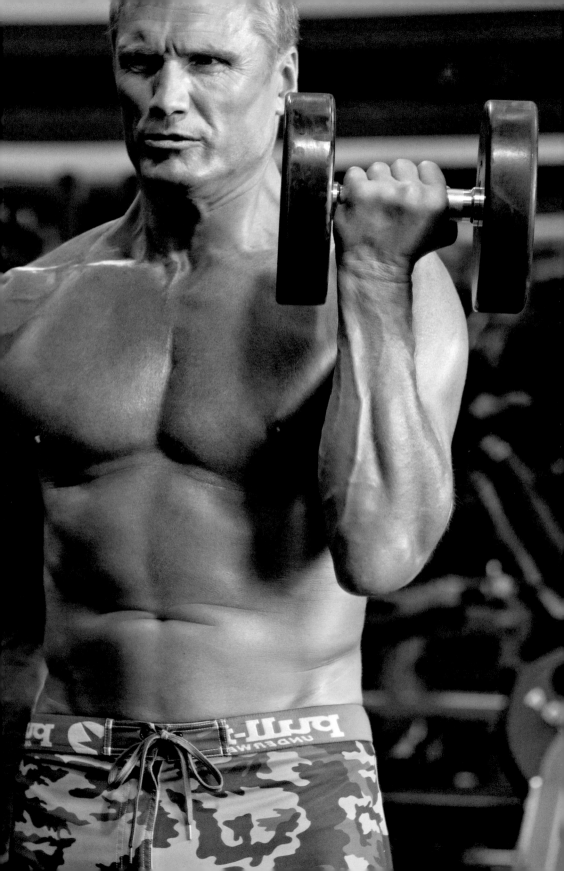

IF THE MASTER IS IRRESISTIBLY DRIVEN TOWARD THIS GOAL, HE MUST SET OUT ON HIS WAY AGAIN, TAKE THE ROAD TO THE ARTLESS ART. HE MUST DARE TO LEAP INTO THE ORIGIN, SO AS TO LIVE BY THE TRUTH AND IN THE TRUTH, LIKE ONE WHO HAS BECOME ONE WITH IT.

HE MUST BECOME A PUPIL AGAIN, A BEGINNER; CONQUER THE LAST AND STEEPEST STRETCH OF THE WAY, UNDERGO NEW TRANSFORMATIONS.

IF HE SURVIVES ITS PERILS, THEN IS HIS DESTINY FULFILLED; FACE TO FACE HE BEHOLDS THE UNBROKEN TRUTH, THE TRUTH BEYOND ALL TRUTHS, THE FORMLESS ORIGIN OF ORIGINS, THE VOID WHICH IS THE ALL; IS ABSORBED INTO IT AND FROM IT EMERGES REBORN.

(*Zen in the Art of Archery*, E. Herrigel, 1953)

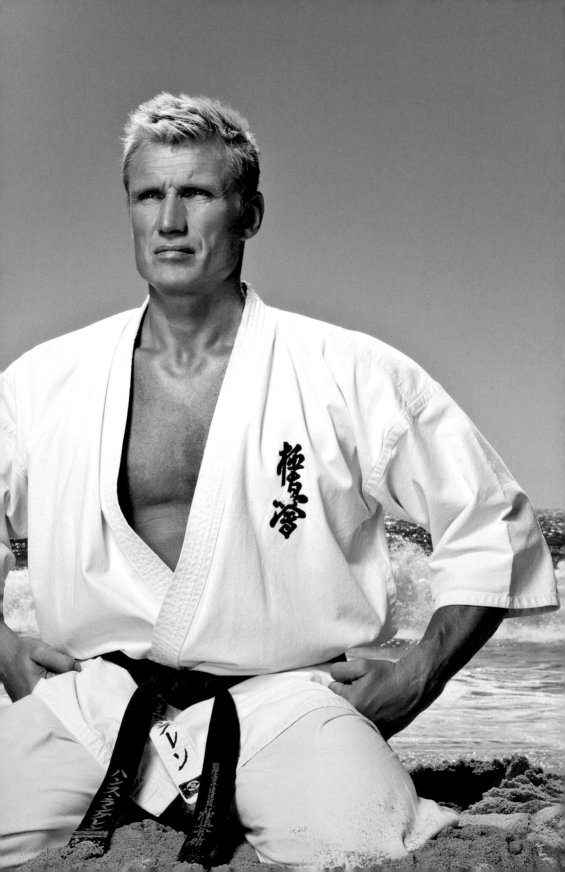

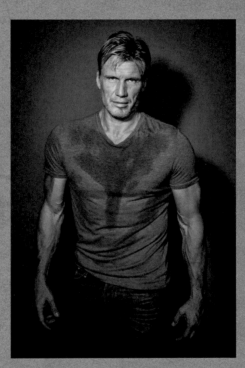

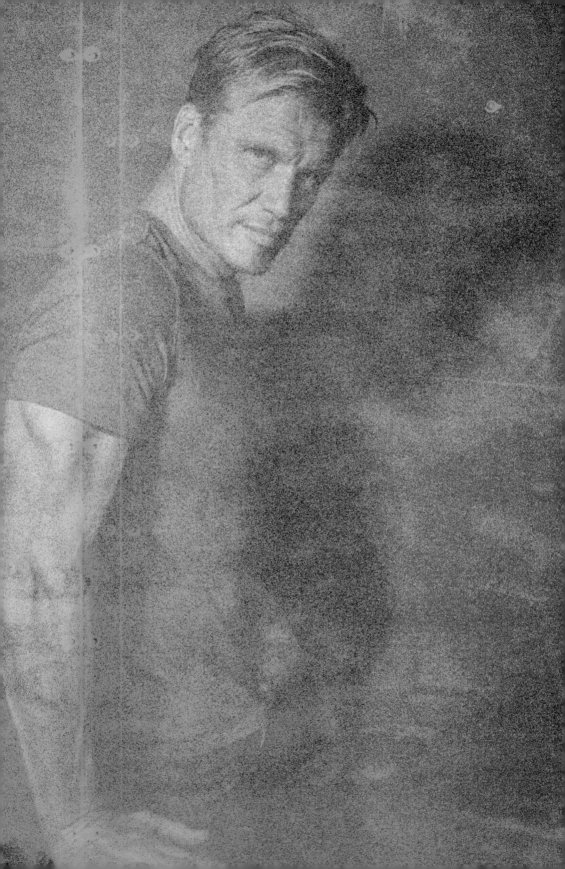

DL PROGRAM 1—OUTLINE

Warm Up (5 minutes)

Abdominals
Hanging leg lifts (3 x 15-20)

Lower back
Back lifts (3 x 20)

Front Thighs
Leg Extension (12/15/10)
Squats or leg press machine (15/12/8/6)
Leg Press—one leg at a time (15 reps per leg)

Chest
Bench press (15/12/8/6)
Dumbbell flyes or cable flyes (2 x 12)

Core
Ball planks/hip rotations with medicine ball
(3 supersets of 45 seconds plank on the balance
ball, 30 seconds rest, 45 seconds seated hip
rotations with medicine ball—rest 30 seconds
between sets)

DL Stretch (3 minutes)

Cardio (3 minutes)

DL PROGRAM 2—OUTLINE

Warm up (5 minutes)

Lower back/Abdominals
Back lifts and v-ups/elbow-to-knees
(3 supersets of 20 reps per exercise)

Hamstrings and buttocks
Deadlifts (15/12/8/6)

Hamstrings
Leg curls (15/12/10)

Calves
Calf raises (3 x 20)

Forearms
Forearm curls (20/15/15: behind the back,
regular curls, reverse curls)

Back
Lat pull-down machine (15/12/8/6)
Seated row machine (2 x 12)
Dumbbell pullovers (15)

DL Stretch (3 minutes)

Cardio (3 minutes)

DL PROGRAM 3—OUTLINE

Warm Up (5 minutes)

Abdominals
Hanging leg lifts (3 x 15-20)

Shoulders
"Arnold" dumbbell press (15/12/10/8)
Combination exercises for shoulders (3 x 12)

Biceps
Standing bicep curls with dumbbells (15/12/10/8)
Concentration curls (2 x 15)

Triceps
Lying triceps press (15/12/10/8)
Triceps press on cable machine (2 x 15)

Lower back/Abdominals
Back lift/sit-ups on the ball (20 resp. 30)

DL stretch (3 minutes)

Cardio (3 minutes)

DL PROGRAM 4—OUTLINE

Exercise bike (3 minutes at low resistance)

Circuit 1
Leg curls (15 reps)
Lat pulls (15 reps)
"Arnold" dumbbell press (15 reps)
Triceps press on the cable machine (15 reps)
Exercise bike (3 minutes at low resistance)

Repeat Circuit 1
Exercise bike (3 minutes at a little higher resistance)

Circuit 2
Leg extensions (15 reps)
Chest press machine (15 reps)
Standing bicep curls with dumbbells (12 reps, left/right)
Upright row (15 reps)
Exercise bike (3 minutes at medium resistance)

Repeat circuit 2
Exercise bike (3 minutes at high resistance)

CIRCUIT 3
Leg press machine (15 reps)
Seated rowing machine (15 reps)
Lateral dumbbell raises (15 reps)
Pec-deck (15 reps)
Exercise bike (3 minutes at high resistance)

Repeat Circuit 3
Rest 2 minutes

Abdominals
Perform this sequence three times without rest:
20 seconds plank,
10 push-ups, 20 seconds side plank on the right side,
10 push-ups,
20 seconds side plank on the left side, 10 push-ups.

DL Stretch (3 minutes)

Cardio (2 minutes shadowboxing)